D0122237

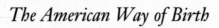

The American Way of Birth

By the same author

HONS AND REBELS

THE AMERICAN WAY OF DEATH

THE TRIAL OF DR SPOCK

THE AMERICAN PRISON BUSINESS

A FINE OLD CONFLICT

THE MAKING OF A MUCKRAKER

FACES OF PHILIP:
A MEMOIR OF PHILIP TOYNBEE

GRACE HAD AN ENGLISH HEART

The American Way
of Birth

JESSICA MITFORD

LONDON
VICTOR GOLLANCZ LTD
1992

First published in Great Britain 1992
by Victor Gollancz Ltd,
14 Henrietta Street, London WC2E 8QJ

© Jessica Mitford 1992

The right of Jessica Mitford to be identified as author
of this work has been asserted by her in accordance with
the Copyright, Designs and Patents Act, 1988

A CIP catalogue record for this book is available
from the British Library

ISBN 0 575 05430 1

Photoset in Great Britain by
Rowland Phototypesetting Ltd, Bury St Edmunds, Suffolk
and printed by St Edmundsbury Press Ltd,
Bury St Edmunds, Suffolk

To
Ted & Peewee Kalman
and their daughter
Janice

with profound gratitude
for their inestimable
help through
a long and difficult labour.

CONTENTS

Part Five: Epilogue

PART ONE

In the Beginning

Chapter 1

INTRODUCTION

It is somehow reassuring to discover that the word 'travel' is derived from 'travail', denoting the pains of childbirth. There is in truth a similarity between the two conditions. Travel can be fraught with aggravating circumstances: unscheduled delays, missed connections, hanging about for hours among strangers in some remote airport, all compounded by your vivid recollections of news accounts detailing the latest spectacular plane crash. Obvious analogies will occur to those who have experienced travail.

However, the rewards soon outweigh the inconveniences – in travel, your eventual arrival at a longed-for destination; in travail, the pleasing sight and sound of a sweet newborn baby. In each case, although thoroughly exhausted, you quickly recover. A curious amnesia takes over in which all memory of the discomforts you have endured is wiped out, and your determination never, ever to do *that* again fast fades.

My own experiences of childbirth, now long ago and mostly far away, seem to have been fairly typical for their time and place.

My first child was born in 1937, when I was twenty and my husband, Esmond Romilly, nineteen. We were living in Bermondsey, a working-class district in London's East End. This was, of course, some years before Britain's postwar National Health Service was established, but the militant Bermondsey branch of the Labour Party, far to the left of the national Labour leadership, had taken these matters into its own hands. Down the road from where we lived was the Labour Party maternity clinic, which furnished free antenatal, or prenatal as it is called in the States, advice, the services of a doctor and nurse to deliver the baby, and free care for the newborn.

Nothing could have gone more smoothly. The doctor and nurse arrived in jig time, minutes after I telephoned to say that my labour had started. Esmond, his knowledge of the husband's role derived from novels and movies, boiled up quantities of water in all available kettles and saucepans while the nurse put down yards of brown paper on my bed to protect it from the messy business ahead.

As the labour pains intensified, the doctor gave me a hand-held gadget consisting of a mask that fitted over the nose and mouth and emitted gas to put you to sleep. Once you were unconscious, your hand fell away until the next pain woke you – at which point you could decide whether or not to help yourself to more gas. To me, that was a perfect system, as it gave the mum-in-travail total control of her situation. I must have been a fairly avid gas guzzler, as I remember little else except the doctor, in all ways the soul of kindness, triumphantly handing me the lovely baby, now all cleaned up with some of Esmond's hot water.

In those days, new mothers were supposed to stay in bed for many days. Each morning and afternoon the Bermondsey district nurse came in to bathe the baby and give me a sponge bath. Sometimes the doctor would stop by on his busy rounds to see how we were doing. I could not have wished for better treatment.

Fast-forward to 1941. I was living in Seminary Hill, Virginia, a community near Washington, DC, with Clifford and Virginia Durr, to whose teeming household I was shortly to add yet another member. Esmond was off in Canada, training for the Royal Canadian Air Force. Virginia Durr, herself the mother of four, insisted that I should go to the hospital for the birth of my baby. I hated that idea – why not have it at home? Absolutely not, said Virginia. All one needs is a quantity of stout brown paper, boiling water, and a competent doctor, I pleaded – but to no avail. She chased me off to a highly touted, fashionable 'obstetrician', a word I'd never heard before. I soon had a dramatic falling-out with him. At each visit, for which he charged $5 – a large amount in those days – he demanded a sample of my urine. To my absolute fury I discovered that Virginia's sister Josephine, wife of Supreme Court Justice Hugo Black, was being treated by the same obstetrician for menopausal troubles

– for which he prescribed injections of the urine of pregnant women at the outrageous cost of $10 per shot. I stormed into his office, accused him of profiteering by selling my urine to Josephine and charging both of us, and told him he was fired forthwith. He seemed astonished, and had nothing to say in his defence.

Eventually, unwilling – and indeed unable – to keep paying $5 for alleged prenatal care, I was accepted in February 1941 as a charity patient at Columbia Hospital, Washington. The anaesthetic given there was unlike anything I'd heard of before or since; possibly a short-lived fad of the moment. It consisted of hot air pumped up one's rectum, rather agony while being administered, but it must have served its purpose, as I remember almost nothing about the actual birth except for the joyful moment when the nurse handed me the baby, wrapped in pink for a girl.

That autumn, Esmond was posted to his Royal Canadian Air Force unit in England. In November 1941, his plane was lost over the North Sea. Two years later, Robert Treuhaft and I were married. We had met in Washington, where Bob was a lawyer with the Office of Price Administration, and we decided to settle in San Francisco. Thereafter my personal experiences of birth took place in California.

By the time my third was born, in 1944, I was thoroughly inured to the idea of going to hospital to have a baby; all my American contemporaries, women in their twenties, were doing it. Anyway, there was no available alternative that I knew of, nothing remotely like the Bermondsey set-up.

At the time, I was working in the San Francisco Office of Price Administration. Once more the prenatal requirement for urine samples. In this respect, the complaint of feminists that male doctors know too little about female anatomy is well borne out: what woman can possibly urinate into that tiny bottle without making a mess all over the lavatory seat? So I went round to my male OPA colleagues, far better equipped for the purpose, soliciting contributions which they cheerfully supplied. I don't think the doctor noticed the difference; in any event, he made no comment.

Come the actual birth, the doctor recommended yet another anaesthetic: this time it was something called a 'caudal block', consisting of an injection into the spine – the idea being to numb you from the waist down so that although fully conscious you would feel nothing of the labour pains. The injection was absolute torture, and so were the headaches that persisted for several days.

Evidently the doctor was well aware of our left-wing proclivities – very likely I had tried to proselytise him during the prenatal visits – because when the baby was finally born, he held it up by its feet and gave it a resounding smack on the bottom, saying, 'One of these progressive kids. I reckon this is the last good spanking he'll ever get.'

In 1947, at the age of thirty, I had my fourth and last child. In those days, friends would look askance at the very idea of having a baby at such a late age: 'Have you considered that by the time it's fifteen, you will be forty-five? Middle-aged? And stuck with bringing up a teenager?'

We had moved to Oakland, and were members of the Permanente Health Plan, which provided cradle-to-grave medical services to participating trade unions and other groups.

Benjamin (for such was his name, meaning, I hoped, youngest and last) was a month late by any reckoning. Eventually my waters broke, supposedly the portent for the onset of labour. We telephoned the hospital and were told to show up there without delay, which we did, to my subsequent regret, for the following three days were fairly unpleasant.

What happened next was – precisely nothing, nary a twinge nor a sign of incipient labour. The only solution, I was told, would be to induce labour via a drug, Pitocin, to be given by injection into one's behind. Every hour on the hour, 'Roll over,' I was instructed, and in would go what appeared to be the longest needle in the history of needles, into alternate buttocks. Fifteen of these per day was the max permitted by medical protocol. Day 1 passed; encouraging pains began, but soon subsided. Ditto on Day 2. By the end of Day 3 I was a veritable pincushion, inert recipient of forty-five injections. Suddenly, after the forty-fifth shot, Benj made his move.

The nurses, having observed that things were getting serious, hurried me into a delivery room and strapped me down on a bed, legs apart, feet secured in iron stirrups, wrists in cuffs – a cruel form of torture – while they summoned a doctor and an anaesthetist. These appeared, but all too briefly; loud shrieks of utter anguish were coming from the adjacent delivery room, so they rushed away to minister to the sufferer. It seemed a bit unfair, as I was sure that my agony could easily match that of my neighbour; but early training of the don't-make-a-fuss-don't-shout-in-public variety lingered on, so that a low, inarticulate moan or two was all I could manage. The nurse explained that as it was now after 6 p.m., dinnertime, all the other doc/anaesthetist teams were off having their supper. (There must be a moral: never give birth between 6 and 8 p.m.) Eventually a doctor did show up, just in time to ease out a huge baby that weighed in at nine and a half pounds. My extreme delight at welcoming the newcomer was only slightly marred by the annoyance of overhearing the doctor telling Bob that it had been a very easy birth.

So much for recollections dredged up from many decades ago. My curiosity about the contemporary American birth scene was first aroused in 1988, by two old friends, Ted and Peewee Kalman, stalwart colleagues of ours in the early days of the civil rights movement. Their daughter Janice, twenty-seven that year, is a lay midwife practising home birth deliveries in Chico, California. The very word 'midwife' had a distinctly old-fashioned ring; hadn't they pretty much disappeared from the scene some fifty years ago? Not so, the Kalmans told me; in many rural areas – Deep South, Midwest, parts of California – midwives were the principal birth attendants in homes of poor people until the 1970s, when they were chased out of their trade by the ever-vigilant medical professional societies. Today, midwifery is making – or trying to make, against considerable odds – a comeback, fuelled by the feminist movement and assorted proponents of a back-to-nature life-style.

Janice had pursued her unusual calling in Chico with great success for a couple of years, during which time her practice had grown and flourished – until in a truly bizarre turn of events she found herself the subject of investigation by the California Board of Medical Quality Assurance with a view to possible criminal prosecution for allegedly practising medicine without a licence. If convicted, she faced a maximum penalty of six months in jail and a $2,000 fine.

Had somebody turned her in to the authorities – a disaffected

mother, or a malicious neighbour? Apparently not; BMQA (pronounced 'Boomqua') had acted on its own. I scented the familiar
aroma of a bureaucracy in the service of special-interest groups,
hunting easy prey.

Wishing to learn more, in January 1989 I went with Janice's
parents to visit her. Chico, two and a half hours' drive north of San
Francisco, is an unprepossessing little town, conservative in outlook
and a perennial butt of Herb Caen, the *San Francisco Chronicle* colum-
nist, who claims that Chico's grocery stores display processed cheese
on their gourmet shelves.

In 1982 Janice, an anthropology major at Pitzer College in Clare-
mont, California, from which she would graduate the following year,
went to Peru on a student field trip. Living for some months in a
remote hamlet, she became friends with the local midwife, a woman
in her sixties, who in long conversations described many a birth she
had attended before Peru became subject to the uncertain blessings
of enlightened modern birth procedures.

'I hung out with the women of the village,' Janice said. 'They told
me about the gradual shift from traditional birth assistants to clinics –
so-called sanitariums – where the younger women go.' From Janice's
description, the local facility should have been called the unsani-
tarium: it was filthy, she said, with unwashed bloody sheets, and
drugs scattered about without supervision as to their use. 'The man
in charge, called the "sanitarian", is a local peasant with perhaps
three months' training.' Did the old midwife still attend births? 'Yes,
mostly those of "kinship", meaning anything from actual relatives to
friends of friends.'

Fascinated by what she had seen in Peru, Janice returned to the
United States, determined to learn midwifery and herself become
a practitioner. (As I have observed in subsequent encounters with
midwives around the country, the decision to embrace this calling
often seems to strike with a force akin to religious conversion.) She
apprenticed with lay midwives in the San Francisco Bay Area, and
later at a birthing centre in El Paso, Texas, where she completed an
intensive clinical and academic course. She finished her training in
New Mexico, passing the state board exam in the top percentile, and

is fully licensed in that state as a 'direct entry', or lay, midwife.

Her lawyer, Paul Persons, filled me in on Janice's legal situation. 'I called the BMQA investigator who told me he would refer her case to the district attorney for prosecution. He admitted to me that although he had contacted several of Janice's clients, he had been unable to find one to make a complaint; and that his sole evidence against her was that she had signed two birth certificates, which he considers proof that she is practising medicine without a licence.'

(Presumably taxi drivers are automatically licensed. One is always reading of some stalwart cabbie who, hurrying to the hospital with a pregnant woman, is too late and himself delivers the mother of a fine eight-pound boy. 'And his middle name is Al, after *me*!' the cabbie proudly tells the avid camera crew on the local TV news. Interestingly, in California a cabdriver may sign a birth certificate with impunity; not so a midwife.)

Should Janice's case come to trial, Persons had a three-pronged defence in mind: (1) normal childbirth is not an illness, or a circum-stance requiring medical intervention; hence, in assisting at home births, Janice was not practising medicine without a licence; (2) as she is a fully licensed lay midwife in the state of New Mexico, the prosecution is in restraint of trade; (3) she had no alternative but to break the law (called the defence of necessity). 'I'd cite the fact that in Chico and environs, there's a whole class of people who don't have health care provisions, don't have insurance, don't qualify for Medi-Cal [California's medical assistance programme for families on welfare] – and tax evaders, who have no proof that they exist!' Persons explained. 'All these could profit greatly from a lay midwife's pro-gramme.'

Janice gave me a rundown on her *modus operandi*. Her fee is $800 per home birth – local obstetricians charge $1,200, to which must be added hospital costs. Her services: eleven prenatal visits of an hour or more in her office; one prenatal house call to make sure that all is in readiness for the birth ('I take a good look around the home to see that the kitchen, bathroom, et cetera, are in sanitary condition; if not, I tell 'em in no uncertain terms that they'll have to clean up before the baby comes!'); attendance at the birth, and three sub-sequent house calls on the mother and newborn; one family-planning session; and unlimited phone consultation. Totting this up, it comes to approximately forty hours per birth, or $20 an hour gross income. 'After paying the rent and phone bill, it's more like five or six dollars per hour,' Janice said ruefully. 'Nobody makes a living at midwifery in California.'

Like most California lay midwives, Janice accepts only 'low-risk' clients. ('We don't refer to them as *patients*,' she told me. 'Patients are ill people, not normal pregnant women.') Taken at face value, 'low-risk' would seem a fairly simple designation for a healthy young woman whose prenatal diagnosis showed no abnormal or unusual features. But who is or isn't high-risk or low-risk is, as I later discovered, a passionately debated subject.

Janice is such an enthusiastic, thoroughly self-confident person, so in love with her work, that it was with some trepidation that I headed into the obvious question that anyone would want to ask: Suppose that, with all systems go and a completely normal birth in progress, at some stage things go seriously wrong – something awful happens? 'In that case,' she answered, 'I transfer the client to hospital, to my back-up obstetrician.' The identity of these back-ups is, she added, a closely held secret; if their names should become known to medical colleagues, they would be subject to ostracism, their hospital privileges and licence to practise in jeopardy.

For a closer look, I spent an evening in Janice's office, a small but commodious house converted for the purpose, an erstwhile bedroom used as the prenatal examination room. A dozen or so people were gathered in the sitting room: young women with babes in arms delivered by Janice; others in various stages of pregnancy (including one woman in early labour whose baby was born the next day); a few husbands; and two midwives, former colleagues of Janice's, who had been chased out of the practice for fear of BMQA.

One of these, Katy, gave me an overview of the midwifery situation in Chico, where she had delivered eighty-five babies in the three years of her tenure. Her clients were of two distinct types: middle-class white women, advocates of an alternative life-style stressing feminist health practices à la *Our Bodies, Ourselves* (the much revised and reprinted women's health guide by the Boston Women's Health Book Collective), and (surprise!) deep conservatives, fundamentalists whose concern is that the father, the man of the family, should be on hand to supervise the birth. About 15 per cent of Katy's cases fit this category, including those who choose home birth for religious reasons: Seventh-Day Adventists, Jehovah's Witnesses, Christian Scientists, and Mormons.

Katy's husband owns a brewery. She reluctantly withdrew from midwifery because no insurance is available to lay midwives; her husband's business could be wiped out if a lawsuit was brought against her. 'There's too much at stake,' she said.

Janice's clients were, I gathered, a fairly prosperous group, their occupations mostly in the middle-income bracket: a manager at McDonald's, an owner of a small bakery, a health education counsellor, a teacher of 'home studies'. What had impelled them to seek out the services of a midwife rather than a trained obstetrician?

Several of them discussed their dire experiences in the hospital with previous births. They described callous and neglectful treatment by the medical staff – being forced to lie immobile for hours on end in the early stages of labour so as not to disturb the foetal monitor strapped to the abdomen, during which time no doctor or nurse came near them. Labour unnecessarily induced for the convenience of the doctor, or unnecessary Caesareans for the same reason. Enormous hospital charges: one woman was charged $800 for a two-hour stay in the hospital; another, $1,200 for a twelve-hour stay, exclusive of the doctor's bill.

The most chilling of all was the account given by Sharon: 'I had a bad experience with my first baby,' she said. 'I had premature labour, the baby was born early – the doctor did an episiotomy which tore into my rectum. It was a horrible experience. I consulted Janice, who agreed to be my midwife for my next birth, on condition that prenatal exams indicated that I would have a normal delivery.' But again, the second baby came early, putting Sharon into the high-risk category. She went to the hospital, where the doctor ordered a sonogram (a method of using ultrasound vibrations to listen to the foetal heart), administered by a technician who reported that the test showed the baby had an 'abnormal head'. Sharon was rushed by ambulance (at a cost of $1,000) to Sacramento, eighty-five miles away, for special care, and her baby was delivered by Caesarean. One day later, the doctors informed her that the diagnosis of the sonogram technician had been wrong; the baby seemed to be quite normal. They arranged for a specialist to see the child – which he did, *one week later*, confirming the good news that the baby was absolutely OK. It does not require much stretch of the imagination to visualise the continuing nightmare, for Sharon, of the ten days that elapsed between sonogram and expert paediatric reassurance as to the well-being of her newborn. Incidentally, the whole caper – ambulance and hospital stay in Sacramento – cost her a cool $11,000, exclusive of the physician's fee.

Throughout the evening at Janice's, listening to conversations around the room, my main impression was one of complete confidence in Janice and her methods, as well as affectionate esteem for her as a friend and mentor, a reliable guide through the uncertain shoals of childbirth.

Shortly after the Chico expedition, I went to visit Dr Patte Coombes in remote Twain Harte, a small village in the foothills of the Sierra. Dr Coombes's position is very different from Janice Kalman's. She is a sixty-three-year-old physician, a general practitioner who in her twenty-three years of practice has delivered some four thousand babies in the two local hospitals and in innumerable home births without a single death of mother or child; nor has she ever been sued for malpractice in connection with her childbirth practice. In a series of secret meetings that she was not permitted to attend, the hospital authorities, led by local obstetricians, voted in July 1987 to revoke her hospital privileges.

How did all this come about? The crux of Dr Coombes's philosophy of childbirth is 'informed freedom of choice' for the mother. For example, if a woman in normal labour balked at being subjected to technological procedures such as the sonogram, Dr Coombes would back her up: 'We know very little about the long-term effects of some of these devices,' she said. Nor would she endorse the use of artificial methods to speed up labour, except in unusual circumstances. Soon she was on a collision course with her obstetrical colleagues.

Hospital protocol mandates that in cases deemed by obstetricians to fall into the high-risk category, an OB consult must be called in by the general practitioner. Conditions automatically considered high-risk by the mainstream obstetrical establishment (although many individual obstetricians strongly disagree) include breech births, twins, unduly prolonged labour, and a previous delivery by Caesarean.

'In each case, I carefully explained to the patient exactly what was involved, and asked her if she wanted me to notify the consult,' said Dr Coombes. 'If she said no, I respected her wishes.'

Ever lurking in the wings was the strong probability that in any of these allegedly high-risk cases, the consult would whisk the patient off for a Caesarean. The hospital's Caesarean rate in any given month ranges from 25 to 33 per cent, Dr Coombes said; her personal rate in 4,000 births was less than five per cent.

Dr Coombes first became aware of the hospital obstetricians' opposition to her methods in the case of a patient who had had a previous C-section (doctor language for Caesarean). 'I was doubtful if a C-section was indicated, and my examination confirmed that vaginal delivery would be successful in this case. While my patient was in labour, and doing fine, I was ordered to have her sign a statement on the letterhead of Sonora Community & Sierra Hospitals.'

The statement, headed 'To Whom It May Concern', requires the patient to acknowledge that she has been informed of hospital policy 'to have a mandatory consult by an OB/GYN specialist' if she is considered to be a high-risk delivery. The punch line: 'I have further been informed that by refusing this consult, I am taking the responsibility of jeopardising my own life, including possible death, along with jeopardising the life of my unborn child, including death.'

Confronted with this positively ghoulish statement, the unhappy patient burst into tears – but she signed. Is this sort of statement usually presented, or was it expressly written for you? I asked Dr Coombes. The latter, she believed.

After revocation of Coombes's hospital privileges on the ground that her work was 'substandard' and 'in flagrant violation of good standards of care', newspaper reporters questioned the hospital authorities about her unblemished record of four thousand births without mishap. Their lame response: 'She was just lucky.'

Reaction of the Twain Harte community was fast and furious. A petition addressed to the hospital with 400 signatures demanded Dr Coombes's reinstatement; the local newspaper, the Sonora *Union Democrat*, ran pictures of a hundred picketers, mostly couples with their Coombes-delivered children, surrounding the hospital. Besides dozens of eloquent letters from satisfied Coombes customers published day after day in the *Union Democrat* and the Modesto *Bee*, Dr Coombes has a huge boxful of loving and supportive letters from former patients.

Of special interest was one from a mother of twins, the subject of a major specific charge against Dr Coombes – failure to summon an obstetrical consult for a high-risk patient. Understandably enraged that her case should have been discussed *in camera*, without her knowledge or permission, by the hospital committee that voted to expel Dr Coombes, the mother wrote to the *Union Democrat*: 'It was the kind of birth I had always wanted. Now six months later I found out that they have formed an ad hoc committee against my doctor questioning the way my birth was handled. I would like to know where my rights come in. No one asked me about it and I was not asked for the hearing.'

The most impressive judgment on the ordeal of Patte Coombes came from far-off Copenhagen in a letter from the World Health Organization, the international health agency of the United Nations, signed by Marsden Wagner, European regional officer for maternal and child health: 'We here in WHO believe very strongly that the type of maternity service which you have been providing is the best type of primary health care that can be provided to women during pregnancy and birth . . . indeed the best epidemiological data suggest that your type of care is in general safer than the hospital-based care typically available in the US.'

These encounters left me with myriad questions. I felt that I had opened at most a tiny crack shedding a minuscule ray of light on the whole vast, intricate American birth scene. For more than that, I would have to seek out obstetricians of both sexes and various views; certified nurse-midwives (now employed in many hospitals, licensed by the states in which they work); lay or direct-entry midwives; and, perhaps most important, the victims and beneficiaries of all the above, viz., people who have had babies.

But I was only at the beginning of a long list of problems and subjects to be considered and investigated. It seemed logical, confronting the complexities of the present, to take first a brief glance at the past. Surely things now couldn't be as bad as they were then?

Chapter 2

A GLANCE BACKWARD

Midwives, from earliest days the traditional attendants at childbirth, were in for very rough times during the late Middle Ages. The major impetus for their persecution was the publication circa 1484 of *Malleus Maleficarum* (in English, *The Hammer of Witches*) by two German Dominican monks, Heinrich Krämer and Jakob Sprenger. Its message was enhanced with a prefatory bull issued by Pope Innocent VIII, who delegated Krämer and Sprenger as inquisitors throughout northern Germany. Furthermore, the *Malleus*, as required reading for all Roman Catholic judges and magistrates, had a large built-in captive readership, what today's publishing industry would consider an author's dream deal; the book became a best-seller throughout Europe.

A few quotes from this immensely long treatise may serve to convey the general viewpoint of the authors.

In Part I, to the question 'Why is it that Women are chiefly addicted to Evil Superstitions?' they answered:

Let us now chiefly consider women; and first, why this kind of perfidy is found more in so fragile a sex than in men . . . specifically with regard to midwives, who surpass all others in wickedness.

Cataloguing the criminal propensities of women, the authors rose to a crescendo of rage:

All wickedness is but little to the wickedness of a woman . . . What else is a woman but a foe to friendship, an unescapable punishment, a necessary evil, a natural temptation, a desirable calamity, a domestic danger, a delectable detriment, an evil of nature painted with fair colours! . . . The root of all woman's vices is avarice . . . When a woman thinks alone, she thinks evil.

Part II provided a description of 'methods by which witchcraft is inflicted, and how it may be auspiciously removed'. This was mostly about various spells cast by witches. Of course, we all know that they could fly through the air at immense speeds (broomsticks, by the way, are not mentioned in the *Malleus*) and could perform various tiresome acts such as causing cows to run dry or harvests to fail.

But oh! Their misdeeds as recorded in the *Malleus* far surpassed any of the above. Talk about dirty tricks! Aside from fornicating with the Devil – a favourite pastime, it seems – they could 'Deprive Man of his Virile Member', 'Change Men into the Shape of Beasts', and 'Inflict Every Sort of Infirmity' including leprosy and epilepsy.

Midwives were the chief culprits: 'Witch midwives cause the greatest damage, either killing children or sacrilegiously offering them to devils . . . The greatest injuries to the Faith are done by midwives; and this is made clearer than daylight itself by the confessions of some who were afterwards burned.'

In Part III we are treated to descriptions of tortures appropriate to different stages of interrogation, to be used in securing a confession. The inquisitor in charge was advised to secure the suspect 'in fetters and iron chains, if it seems good to him; and in this matter we leave the conduct of the affair to his own conscience'.

During the questioning, 'let her be often and frequently exposed to torture, beginning with the most gentle of them. And while this is being done, let the Notary write it all down, how she is tortured and what questions are asked and how she answers.' Next, 'if after being fittingly tortured she refuses to confess the truth, he should have other engines of torture brought before her, and tell her she will have to endure these if she does not confess'.

The pioneering work of these holy men soon bore fruit in the shape of wholesale burnings at the stake of accused witches throughout Europe, a craze that over two centuries spread from Germany to Italy, France and eventually to England. According to Barbara

Ehrenreich and Deidre English in *For Her Own Good*, executions averaged six hundred a year for certain German cities; nine hundred witches were destroyed in one year in the Würzburg area; in 1585, two villages in the Bishopric of Trier were left with but one female inhabitant each. Some writers have estimated the total number killed in the millions; more recent assessments have set the figure at a mere 50,000 poor, illiterate peasant women who served as healers and midwives to their neighbours.

One might be inclined to dismiss the macabre work of Krämer and Sprenger and its murderous aftermath as products of deranged medieval minds – fascinating to read as ancient history, but with no particular relevance to modern times – were it not for the introduction by their co-religionist, Rev. Montague Summers, to the 1948 edition of the *Malleus*. His summing up:

> In fine, it is not too much to say that *The Malleus Maleficarum* is among the most important, wisest, and weightiest books of the world . . . One turns to it again and again with edification and interest.

To Rev. Summers, 'it seems plain that the witches were a vast political movement, an organised society which was antisocial and anarchical, a world-wide plot against civilisation'. He entreated his readers to 'approach this great work with open minds and grave intent', and to 'duly consider the world of confusion, of Bolshevism, of anarchy and licentiousness all around today'.

Commenting on the Krämer/Sprenger bias against women in general, Rev. Summers tended to approve, and explained why. Conceding that the 'misogynic trend of various passages' may seem amazing to modern readers, he wrote:

> However, exaggerated as these may be, I am not altogether certain that they will not prove a wholesome and needful antidote in this feministic age, when the sexes seem confounded, and it appears to be the chief object of many females to ape the man, an indecorum by which they not only divest themselves of such charm as they might boast, but lay themselves open to the sternest reprobation in the name of sanity and commonsense.

Having had my fill of Rev. Summers's loony observations, in search of actual 'sanity and commonsense' I went to the November 1990 premiere of *The Burning Times*, a remarkable historical documentary produced and directed by Montreal film-maker Donna Read.

Onscreen, I saw blow-ups of medieval woodcuts showing women in chains being dragged into the flames by robed priests, interspersed with pastoral scenes of the hamlets where women healers were hunted down by the inquisitors. Voice-over commentaries by several historians and scholars described the economic, political, and religious background against which the 'women's holocaust' took place.

Politically, the film told the viewer, the Church was determined to consolidate its hegemony over the peasantry by stamping out all vestiges of customs, some deriving from pagan times, that honoured women as seers, diviners, and healers. The timing of the wholesale burnings coincided with the rise of male medical practitioners trained in Church-controlled universities. Only men were allowed by the Church to become doctors, and it was often their testimony at Inquisition tribunals that sealed the fate of midwives, sending them to a fiery death at the stake.

I asked Donna Read if she perceived any sort of historical parallel between the medieval witch-hunts and today's unremitting efforts by the medical establishment to drive midwives out of their profession. Not exactly a parallel, she said: 'It's more a continuum.' Her purpose in making the film, she told me, was to trace the story of the witch-hunts from the point of view of the victims, to which end she enlisted the help of medievalist scholars in Canada and the United States. Because the only surviving records of the period – and there are precious few of them – were kept by Church officials, research presented enormous problems. Yet the message came through loud and clear; as Donna Read said, 'History is written by the winners.'

Despite the horrors inflicted by the Inquisition on European midwives (which horrors, incidently, never reached such heights in England), the traditional mode of childbirth, with female midwives in attendance, continued unchanged until the late Middle Ages. In the fifteenth to seventeenth centuries there arose a cloud no bigger than a man's hand (it was, in fact, a man's hand), the harbinger of momentous changes to come.

Among the significant developments were the entry into the birth chamber of male practitioners, via the Guild of Barber-Surgeons and university-trained physicians, and the invention in 1588 of childbirth forceps, the first glimmering of the use of technology in this field. The barber-surgeons were constantly embroiled with midwives, whom they sought to displace, and with upper-class university-trained members of the Royal College of Physicians (incorporated in 1518 under a charter granted by Henry VIII), who scorned the barber-surgeons as uneducated quacks.

The barber-surgeons, as their name suggests, were adept at cutting hair and shaving beards, and they also brought their sharp knives into use for bloodletting and dentistry. Artisans 'of the urban lower class', according to a class-conscious English writer, they were first chartered in 1376, and incorporated as the Company of Barber-Surgeons by Edward IV in 1461. They were granted a coat of arms and later were immortalised by Holbein in a picture showing King Henry VIII giving a charter to the barber-surgeons, who wore 'gowns of rich stuff, red and black hoods, some in coifs'.

Like other guilds of the period, the barber-surgeons required members to swear an oath agreeing to abide by guild rules and to be loyal to the city. The guild master was charged with upholding morals and standards, and after 1614 held yearly dissections and anatomy lectures, which members were obliged to attend.

Enter the Chamberlen family, eccentric, avaricious, belligerent, and extremely clannish. They were Huguenots, natives of Paris who in 1569 fled the Roman Catholic onslaught against their Protestant co-religionists to settle in London, where they plied their trade as barber-surgeons. There, circa 1588, Peter Chamberlen perfected his amazing invention, childbirth forceps.

Until the advent of forceps, there had been no live deliveries of births presenting unusual difficulties. Instead, to save the mother's life, various hooks and a nightmarish instrument called a cranioclast were used to break open the child's skull, dismember it, and drag it out bit by bit. (There was, however, spiritual comfort for the true believer in a 'syringe for baptism *in utero*'. This was roughly shaped to fit the birth canal, was filled with holy water, and presumably would have been brought into service just before the cranioclast was produced to perform its lethal mission.)

The Chamberlen device was actually rather simple, and may have been adapted by the clever Chamberlen gang from the practice of some midwives who used spoons to facilitate birth. It consisted of oversized hollow metal spoons with handles that could be inserted separately, then joined and locked together so that the spoons cupped the baby's head to draw it out.

One might suppose that the Chamberlens would have been anxious to broadcast the grand news of their lifesaving invention and to share it with fellow birth attendants – midwives and physicians. Far from it; these grasping tightwads, bent only on their own enrichment, kept the forceps a closely held family secret for over a hundred years.

The Chamberlen brothers, confusingly both named Peter – Peter the Elder being the forceps inventor – travelled round England, charging enormous fees, always payable in advance, for attending births. The forceps were concealed in a richly carved locked casket. The brothers went to amazing lengths to prevent information about their instrument from leaking out. Contrary to the custom of the day, they excluded female family members from the delivery chamber; they blindfolded the labouring woman; and to confound the anxious relatives still further, they made all sorts of diversionary noises such as ringing loud bells, rattling chains, and banging with hammers during the delivery.

The wildly fluctuating fortunes of this bizarre family over several generations must have been for them a veritable roller-coaster ride, full of soaring ups and thudding downs.

Peters Elder and Younger were in constant hot water with the Company of Barber-Surgeons, to which they both belonged. The annals of the company from 1599 to 1601 record failure to pay dues – 'severall arrearages of their debtes to this house' – and absence from the obligatory lectures.

They also fell afoul of the College of Physicians, who accused

Peter the Elder of practising medicine '*illicita mala*', also known as '*malpraxis*', and in 1609 fined him forty shillings for this offence. Three years later, the college (which was empowered under its charter to imprison those it found guilty of malpractice) sent him to Newgate prison for a similar transgression of their rules prohibiting anyone but a physician from dispensing medicine.

This became an important test case for the barber-surgeons seeking the right to prescribe medicine to their patients. P. the Elder fought back and persuaded the Lord Mayor of London to intercede on his behalf – to no avail; the physicians stood their ground. So he went up the social scale and appealed to the Archbishop of Canterbury, who, at the request of the Queen, obtained his release. (This did not deter P. the Younger, ever-loyal brother, from slanging the physicians, for it is recorded in the minutes of the college for November 1613 that 'Dr Fludd complained that Peter the Younger had used most insolent language against myself and others, members of the College.')

In due course, Peter the Younger married and begat a son named Peter – what else? – who studied medicine abroad and in 1628 was elected a fellow of the College of Physicians. Dr Peter Chamberlen, like his father and uncle a rambunctious type, seems to have been an early hippie, 'gravely admonished' by the college 'to change his mode of dress and no longer follow the frivolous fashion of the youth at Court, but adopt the decent and sober dress of the members of the College'.

A few years after Dr Peter's election to the College of Physicians, in 1634, he petitioned the King to establish a Corporation of Midwives, naming himself as governor. The midwives retaliated with their own petition, referred by the King to the Archbishop of Canterbury and the Bishop of London, who were empowered to license midwives;

> Neither can Dr Chamberlane* teach the art of midwifery in most births because he hath no experience in itt but by reading and it must bee continuall practice in this kind that will bringe experience.

---

* Spelling varies from writer to writer.

The petition further stated:

> Dr Chamberlain's work and the work belonging to midwives are contrary one to the other for he deliv's none without the use of instruments by extraordinary violence in desperate occasions, which women never practised nor desyred for they have neither parts nor hands for that art.

The midwives' case was reinforced by a pronouncement of the College of Physicians to the effect that

> it being true that is reported by the Midwifes, Dr Chamberlane doth often refuse to come to the poor, they not being able to pay him according to his demands and for the rich he denies them his help until he hath first bargained for great rewards which besides that they are in themselves dishonest covetous and unconscionable courses, they are also contrary to the laws and statutes of our College to which by Oath he is bound.

Dr Peter lost that round. The Bishops condemned his behaviour and, rubbing salt in the wound, further decreed that he should 'forthwith bee a Suitor to the Lord Bishopp of London for a Lycense to practize the Art of Midwifery'. Years later, still bent on revenge (the Chamberlens were an unforgiving lot), Dr Peter castigated the midwives in a pamphlet entitled *A Voice in Rhama: or, the Crie of Women and Children* (1647), in which he denounced 'Ignorance and Disorder amongst some uncontrolled femal-Arbiters [sic] of Life and Death'.

In spite of the opprobrium heaped upon them by their contemporaries from physicians to midwives, the Chamberlen tribe continued to flourish like so many green bay trees. Their fame, and news of their great invention, travelled throughout Europe; they were summoned to the birth chambers of nobility and royalty. The epitaph of Dr Peter Chamberlen, who died in 1683 at the ripe age of eighty-two, records that he served as 'Physician in ordinary to three Kings and Queens of England, viz. King James and Queen Anne, King Charles ye First and Queen Mary, King Charles ye Second and Queen Katherine, and also to some foreign Princes, having travelled to most parts of Europe, and speaking most of the languages'. And in 1688 his son, Dr Hugh Chamberlen Senior, was called by King James II to officiate at the birth of his son, best known to history as the Old Pretender.

Eventually the miraculous forceps were sold by Dr Hugh Chamberlen to a Dutchman in Amsterdam. According to Logan Clendening, 'the negotiations are very obscure, and at this late date we cannot tell exactly what happened, except that it looks like dirty work at the crossroads'. No surprises here, just what one would expect from a Chamberlen. The precious casket, when opened years later, proved to contain a useless metal object, bearing no resemblance to forceps.

In another account, the original forceps were found in 1813 under the floor of a closet by a lady (unnamed) 'in a curious chest or cabinet' that contained various oddments – old coins, trinkets, gloves and many letters from Dr Chamberlen to members of his family – and the forceps. These were eventually presented to the Medico-Chirurgical Society of London.

Who knows the truth of it? – not that it matters, for by the early eighteenth century numerous doctors had themselves independently tumbled to the idea of forceps, designs for which thereafter proliferated.

The last word is that of Dr Hugh Chamberlen Senior, who in 1672 offered 'an Apology for not publishing the Secret':

> My Father, Brothers, and my Self (tho none else in Europe that I know) have, by God's Blessing, and our Industry, attained to, and long practised a way to deliver Women in this case, without any prejudice to them or their Infants; tho all others (being obliged, for want of such an Expedient, to use the common way) do, and must endanger, if not destroy one or both, with Hooks. By this manual Operation may be dispatched (when there is the least difficulty) with fewer pains, and in less time, to the great advantage, and without danger, both of Woman and Child.

It is a relief to turn from this repulsive family to a practitioner of midwifery whose groundbreaking discovery heralded the end of a principal cause of maternal death: childbed, or puerperal, fever. In contrast to the Chamberlens, Dr Ignaz Semmelweis (1818–1865) immediately disseminated his findings throughout the medical community, and in doing so both published *and* perished. He was driven out of his post at the Vienna Lying-In Hospital, where he had succeeded in virtually eliminating the disease, by an envious and vengeful superior. Dr Semmelweis returned to his native Budapest, where he eventually went mad and died in an insane asylum.

Dr Semmelweis's analysis of the cause and cure of childbed fever is, in hindsight, breathtakingly simple. The cause: doctors and medical students would come directly from the hospital morgue, where they had performed autopsies on victims of the fever, to the maternity ward, where they would poke their dirty fingers up the vaginas of women in labour. The cure: wash your hands! and voilà, the death rate from this horrible disease plummeted.

The Vienna Lying-In Hospital was divided into two separate sections: the First Clinic, where medical students received training and tuition in their profession, and the Second Clinic, staffed entirely by midwives. Dr Semmelweis was appointed assistant physician to the First Clinic at the age of twenty-eight, in 1846.

He soon became absorbed in the study of puerperal fever, an obsession that lasted to the end of his life. The horrifying facts were that deaths from the fever in the First Clinic exceeded those in the Second Clinic by more than four to one. Women who delivered on the hospital steps or in the corridors never contracted the disease. Women in tears came pleading to be assigned to the midwives of the Second Clinic and spared the charnel house of the First.

Reasoning empirically (this was some twenty years before Joseph Lister propounded the uses of antiseptics in surgery), Dr Semmelweis decreed that medical students under his jurisdiction should wash their hands in chloride of lime solution on returning from dissecting corpses. Furthermore, he required them to wash their hands after each examination of women in the ward, and to this end arranged for washbasins to be placed strategically between the rows of beds.

The results of this regimen were spectacular. At the end of seven months, Semmelweis announced that deaths from the fever in the First Clinic had dropped from twelve to three per cent. During the next year only one per cent of First Clinic patients died; and from March to December 1848 there was not a single death from the fever.

There were antecedents. Although puerperal fever was known to the ancients, there were few deaths before the establishment of lying-in hospitals and the introduction of procedures requiring manual examination of women in labour.

Throughout the eighteenth century, doctors had wrestled with this terrible epidemic which killed off multitudes of women. The sufferers died in agony, high fever followed by delirium and certain death.

Early on, some of the more alert practitioners observed that the fever was prevalent only in maternity wards, and that somehow dirty conditions in the wards may have been responsible. For example, Dr John Clarke (1761–1815) recapitulated some observations of his predecessors about the history of the disease, first recorded in 1760, eleven years after the establishment of lying-in hospitals, when puerperal fever was 'epidemical in London'. Dr Clarke wrote:

> In the year 1773, the puerperal fever appeared in the lying-in ward of the Royal Infirmary of Edinburgh . . . It began about the end of February, when almost every woman, as soon as she was delivered, or perhaps about twenty-four hours after, was seized with it; and all of them died, though every method was used to cure the disorder. This disease did not exist in the town.

Other medical writers noted the same phenomenon, i.e., the mysterious spread of the fever in hospitals but not in the town, where women gave birth at home. This led to the conclusion that the ailment was contagious. In 1781, Dr Alexander Hamilton (1739–1802) wrote that the childbed fever

> is remarkably infectious . . . like the plague, few escape of those affected . . . It raged in the public hospitals of Paris, London and Dublin, communicating from one person to another with astonishing rapidity, and its ravages were equally striking.

And a French physician, Auguste César Baudeloque (1795–1851), commenting on the introduction of the hand and use of instruments in the birth canal, pondered in his supercilious Gallic fashion:

It would be curious to ascertain in what proportion the disease has declared itself with the number of accouchements effected by the interference of art.

In which conjecture, it turns out, he was absolutely on target.

A peculiar characteristic of puerperal fever was a disgusting smell, called by the medical men a 'foul odour', that emanated from the dying women and permeated the entire ward, lingering in bedclothes, carpets, curtains, and the clothing of the attending physician. Some thought that the smell itself caused the spread of infection. Dr Charles White (1728–1813), Fellow of the Royal College of Surgeons, surgeon and man-midwife of Manchester, in 1773 published his pioneering 'Treatise on the Management of Pregnant and Lying-in Women', which contained the first clearcut statement of the necessity of absolute cleanliness in the lying-in wards. He devoted a long paragraph to specific directions for supplying fresh bed linen, washing carpets, providing plenty of ventilation via open windows – and, above all, isolating the fever victim.

Other doctors followed suit, calling for a virtual spring-cleaning after a patient died of the fever: washing and even painting walls, anything to get rid of the 'miasma' and smell that seemed to spread the infection. Whether these eminently sensible directives were actually carried out, we don't know. In any event, the fever continued to ravage maternity patients until Dr Semmelweis came forward with the definitive answer.

It seems, then, that a good deal of washing did in fact take place pre-Semmelweis; however, as one doctor wrote, 'everyone . . . knows full well that it is almost impossible to remove the smell from the hands for many hours, even with the aid of repeated washing'. Dr Semmelweis's addition to the washing water of chlorine, a recently discovered disinfectant, made the crucial difference. Had chlorine been available in Lady Macbeth's day, she might have had better luck getting rid of the damned spot.

Examples of 'iatrogenic disease', meaning illness caused by doctors, abound in the annals of medicine. Surely puerperal fever is a classic case in point. As Dr Cutter graphically put it in his *History of Midwifery*,

Semmelweis proved with startling clearness and by means of incontrovertible evidence that the examining finger could and did convey infection in the puerperal woman ... His proof of the fatal role of the foul examining finger was an all-important discovery.

In America, the illustrious Dr Oliver Wendell Holmes (1809–1894) was the first of his profession to recognise that puerperal fever was a contagion spread by doctors. Anticipating Semmelweis's findings by a few years, in 1843 Holmes read a paper at a meeting of the Boston Society for Medical Improvement in which he presented evidence based on the experience of colleagues that certain doctors were carrying a contagious presence from patient to patient; and he went so far as to advise doctors to cease practice when they or their patients became ill with the fever.

This put the cat amongst the pigeons. Although his Boston audience was deeply impressed and urged him to publish his thesis (which he did, under the title 'The Contagiousness of Puerperal Fever' in the *New England Quarterly Journal of Medicine and Surgery*, April 1843), other physicians reacted with vitriolic fury.

Holmes's main adversaries were two Philadelphia physicians, Dr Charles D. Meigs (1792–1869) and Dr Hugh L. Hodge (1796–1873), both well known and highly regarded throughout the profession. This battle of the titans was joined in the pages of medical journals and monographs. At issue was the very notion that doctors, prototypical gentlemen and scholars, could themselves be the cause of disease in their patients.

In his article 'On the Non-contagious Character of Puerperal Fever' (Philadelphia, 1852) Dr Hodge exhorted his colleagues

to divest your minds of the overpowering dread that you can ever become, especially to women ... the minister of evil; that you can ever convey, in any possible manner, a horrible virus so destructive in its effects ... as that attributed to puerperal fever.

He advanced the further proposition that it would be most harmful to a woman enduring the stress of birth to add to her troubles the 'cruel, very cruel' suggestion that her trusted doctor might bring deadly contagion: 'It is far more humane ... to keep her happy in ignorance of danger.'

Dr Meigs attacked Holmes with double doses of venom for

> propagating a vile, demoralizing superstition as to the nature and causes of many diseases ... I prefer to attribute them to accident or Providence ... I have practiced midwifery for many long years ... I have made many researches of childbed fever ... Still, I certainly never was the medium of its transmission.

He particularly resented Holmes's suggestion that doctors' dirty hands might be a factor in spreading the disease, as doctors were gentlemen, and gentlemen's hands were clean.

In rebuttal, Holmes cited the case of Dr James Y. Simpson of Edinburgh, who had reported attending the dissection of two cases in which he handled the infected parts. 'His next four childbed patients were affected with fever and it was the first time he had seen it in his practice. As Dr Simpson is a *gentleman*, and as a gentleman's hands are clean, it follows that a gentleman with clean hands can carry the disease.'

Years later, long after the controversy within the medical community had been resolved in his favour, Dr Holmes looked back on it in a letter dated May 8, 1883, to a friend, the librarian of the Boston Medical Library:

> I thought I had proved my point ... I thought I had laid down rules which promised to ensure the safety of the lying-in woman from disease and death carried to her unconsciously by her professional attendant.
>
> Still, I was attacked in my stronghold by the two leading professors of obstetrics in this country.
>
> I defended my position with new facts and arguments and not without rhetorical fervor, at which, after cooling down for half a century, I might smile if I did not remember how intensely and with what good reason my feelings were kindled into the heated atmosphere of superlatives ...
>
> But I think I shrieked my warning louder and longer than any of them, and I am pleased to remember that I took my ground on

the existing evidence before the little army of microbes was
marched up to support my position.

With the start of Queen Victoria's reign in 1837, the growing
demand by upper-class women in both England and America for the
services of male physicians, coupled with the elevation of womanly
modesty to one of the supreme virtues, must have caused many a
conflicting emotion to rage within the feminine breast. Babies were
customarily delivered from under the voluminous skirts of the
mother, her private parts thus shielded from prying masculine eyes.
This procedure must have been more than a little awkward for everyone involved, and hardly conducive to the further enlightenment of
doctors as to the realities of female anatomy.

A prime example of the fatal combination of medical ignorance
and female prudery was the appalling fate of Lady Flora Hastings, a
lady-in-waiting to the Queen's mother.

Victoria loathed 'that odious Lady Flora', as she called her, so it
was with undisguised glee that in February 1839 she reported to
Lord Melbourne, the Prime Minister, that she and her German
governess, Baroness Lehzen, had noticed suspicious changes in Lady
Flora's figure and had concluded that 'there is no doubt that she is
– to use plain words – *with child!!*' The Queen, barely twenty years
old, would presumably have been kept ignorant in general of the
Facts of Life; yet she seemed to be aware that the state of pregnancy
required the active participation of a man. Her candidate for the
deflowerer of Lady Flora was a political enemy, Sir John Conroy,
'Monster and Demon Incarnate', as the Queen wrote in her diary.

The court physician, Sir James Clark, agreed with Victoria's diagnosis. In his scientific fashion he gave his professional opinion that
'nobody could look at Lady Flora and doubt it'. Later, he attended
her for her complaint of biliousness (for she was indeed very ill) and
on several occasions examined her while she was fully dressed. As
gossip about her scandalous condition spread, he asked to examine
her without her clothes, which she indignantly refused.

Eventually, Lady Flora caved in and submitted to a medical examination by two doctors, Sir James Clark and Sir Charles Clarke, a
physician she had known since childhood, thus exposing herself (in

the words of a contemporary) to 'dreadful mortification, and much indelicate inquiry'.

The doctors certified that she was a virgin, but this was not, said Sir Charles, incontrovertible proof of her innocence, as he had heard of cases of virgins becoming pregnant. Needless to say, this interesting observation merely served to intensify Palace speculation about the man responsible – which was ended only after Lady Flora's death in July 1839, five months after the Queen and Baroness Lehzen had first voiced their suspicions to the Prime Minister. An autopsy revealed a huge tumour as the cause of the swelling. The Hastings family was livid; there was talk of duels; the press weighed in with daily diatribes against the Queen, who was hissed by her erstwhile loyal subjects when she ventured forth to the Ascot races.

A tidal wave of female modesty soon made its way across the Atlantic. American obstetricians exhorted one another to be aware of 'the sense of delicacy, on the part of the female', as in the *Obstetrical Catechism*, 1854. First, the doctor should obtain permission from the husband or a 'matronly female' for a hands-on examination. Having done so, 'the room should be darkened, and the patient lightly dressed, and placed in the suitable position'. A third person should be present.

> Q: What is the rule for carrying the hand under the coverings?
> A: The clothes should be properly raised at their lower edges, by the left hand, and then the right hand with the index finger lubricated, passed cautiously up the clothes without uncovering the patient.

Compared to the traditional midwife, who would have been thoroughly familiar with the ins and outs of the female body, and would know where to look and what to look for at various stages of labour, the male practitioner – his knowledge largely derived from textbooks and academic lectures on anatomy – may often have felt woefully inadequate to the task at hand. If so, it was important to conceal this from the patient. An 1848 manual stressed the importance of a reassuring bedside manner, of making 'a good impression in advance', combining 'refined delicacy ... warm sympathy and kind consideration, thus soothing her scruples and enlisting her gratitude. He must also appear perfectly self-possessed under all circumstances, and then she will have full confidence in his skill and judgment.' When passing the lubricated finger under the bedclothes, 'he can proceed with the examination as if it were a simple ordinary proceeding. By exhibiting no hurry, and appearing to think it nothing unusual or in any way strange, the female herself will cease to think so and will not be flurried or shocked.'

The above instructions would have applied only to doctors attending home births, for it goes without saying that in the nineteenth century, in America as well as England, the rich, the middle-class and even the poor-but-genteel would not have dreamed of going to a hospital for the purpose. Maternity wards, rightly regarded as hellholes of infection and death at least until the 1880s, when the spectre of childbed fever had largely subsided, were frequented only by the poorest of the poor: recent immigrants, unmarried girls, homeless women.

These unfortunates, physician fodder one might call them, became subjects of examination and experimentation by doctors, often accompanied by a phalanx of medical students. They were hardly in a position to insist on respect for female modesty, or to object to serving as 'material' (the term of a nineteenth-century obstetrician) in the ever-escalating use of forceps and other experimental devices. How many perished from the ministrations of the medical fraternity, and how many survived, is unknown, there being no statistics on the subject.

There are, however, plentiful records of the fame, acclaim, and fortune amassed by some of the experimenters. Foremost amongst these was Dr James Marion Sims (1813–1883), who started out in 1835 at the age of twenty-two as a country doctor in Alabama and eventually became, according to his own estimate, the second wealthiest of all American physicians. He was hailed by students at Harvard Medical School as 'one of the immortals'; travelled to Europe to attend the Empress Eugénie, the Crown Princess of Saxony, and the Duchess of Hamilton; became president of the American Medical Association; was known by medical historians as 'the Architect of the Vagina'; and saw a statue of himself erected in Central Park by grateful New York matrons.

How did Sims achieve these dizzying heights of wealth, professional recognition, and international renown? He seems to have been endowed with the generic qualities of nineteenth-century self-made American men, the legendary robber barons: single-minded pursuit of his goals, unflagging energy, relentless use of available human resources – and, above all, a total lack of compunction about his exploitation of those less fortunately placed.

In Montgomery, the young Dr Sims began to specialise in disorders of the female organs. He was particularly drawn to one of the more horrible diseases, for which at the time there was no known cure: vesico-vaginal fistulae, tears in the walls between the vagina and bladder that occurred during childbirth, often the result of a badly botched forceps delivery. This caused continual leakage from the bladder. Thousands of women suffered from this condition, which rendered them not only life-long invalids but social pariahs, as the smell from the seepage was intolerable.

In pursuit of a cure, the future Architect of the Vagina bought from their owners several black female slaves afflicted with the sickness, whom he housed in a hut in his back yard. 'I kept all these negroes at my own expense all the time,' he wrote later. 'This was an enormous tax for a young doctor.' (And enormously taxing, no doubt, for the recipients of his bounty.) For four long years, from 1845 to 1849, he operated on Lucy, Betsy, Anarcha, and others – more than thirty times on Anarcha alone, without anaesthetic. The pain must have been almost unendurable; as Dr Sims wrote, 'It was far harder to operate on white women than on negroes.' In one such effort, 'The pain was so terrific that Mrs H. could not stand it and I was foiled completely.'

The operations on the slaves were unrelieved failures; each time, the stitches became infected and the fistulae remained open. Finally, Dr Sims won through by using silver sutures, which did not become infected. He called these 'the greatest surgical achievement of the nineteenth century'.

Having surmounted this formidable hurdle, Sims went from triumph to triumph – there was no stopping him. He forsook

Montgomery for the greater challenge of New York, and in 1855 helped to found the Woman's Hospital, where there was no lack of experimental material. His patients were for the most part destitute Irish immigrants, whom he kept there indefinitely. One of these, Mary Smith, endured thirty operations between 1856 and 1859, just as the slave Anarcha had before her. Dr Sims could now command stupendous fees from his private patients, on whom he conferred the benefits of his experimental successes.

As for Anarcha, Mary Smith, and all those other luckless subjects, there is no telling what became of them.

A dramatic breakthrough, which would transform the childbirth experience for the upper classes, was the discovery in 1847 by Dr James Young Simpson, professor of midwifery at Edinburgh University, of the anaesthetic properties of chloroform. To try it out, on November 4 of that year he invited some medical colleagues to partake of the drug and test its effects. It was a howling success. As he described the occasion to his daughter Eve, 'The first night we took it, Dr Duncan, Dr Keith and I all tried it simultaneously, and were all "under the table" in a minute or two.' When he awoke, the daughter wrote, Dr Simpson 'noted that he was prostrate on the floor and that among the friends about him there was both confusion and alarm. Dr Duncan was snoring heavily, and Dr Keith kicking violently at the table above him. They made several more trials of it that eventful evening and were so satisfied with the results that the festivities did not terminate till a late hour, 3 a.m.'

Dr Simpson was evidently something of a card. He would take vials of chloroform along to dinner parties and press them on fellow guests, causing hilarity all around as the diners fell unconscious and tumbled about on the floor. His sister had a horror of chloroform; he used to threaten her with it, and 'when she fled he gave chase, but she always escaped, for fits of laughter used to seize him and choke him off the pursuit'.

On November 8, four days after the festive evening of the initial testing, Simpson used chloroform in the delivery of the wife of a fellow physician. She was evidently delighted, for she christened her baby daughter, the first child born under chloroform, 'Anaesthesia'

– a pretty enough name for a girl. (Eve Simpson tells us that a Russian boy, first in his country to be vaccinated, was named Vaccinoff. And what of modern medical terms? Somehow names like CaesariAnna for a girl, or Episio Tommy for a boy, have not thus far caught on.)

From the portentous evening of November 4, 1847, to the end of that year, the energetic Dr Simpson gave lectures, wrote pamphlets, and administered chloroform to his numerous grateful maternity patients, all the while (one likes to think) enjoying a greatly enhanced social life, his entertaining after-dinner act doubtless being much in demand.

However, there was trouble ahead. Although the discovery of chloroform was widely hailed by the medical profession as a tremendous boon for use in surgery, for the first time allowing a wretched sufferer to have a limb amputated while sound asleep, its use in childbirth was another matter.

Fellow physicians, and above all the clergy, were soon in hot pursuit of Dr Simpson. Debate pro and con raged in *The Lancet* (then, as now, Britain's foremost medical journal), and the Church of England stood united in opposition, citing Biblical authority that woman should suffer in childbirth as atonement for Eve's original sin. As one clergyman put it, chloroform was 'a decoy of Satan, apparently offering itself to bless woman; but in the end it will harden society, and rob God of the deep earnest cries which arise in time of trouble for help'.

In a swift counter-offensive, aimed at both the clergy and his medical opponents, Dr Simpson published his 'Answer to Religious Objections' in December 1847, one month after his discovery of chloroform. The canny Scotsman pointed out that God Himself was by no means averse to the use of anaesthesia on appropriate occasions, and he quoted Genesis 2:21: 'And the Lord God caused a deep sleep to fall upon Adam, and he slept; and He took one of his ribs, and closed up the flesh instead thereof.'

Given the united opposition of the Church, joined by influential voices in the medical profession, the embattled Dr Simpson may have been apprehensive for the future of the use of chloroform in childbirth. Help was at hand from an unexpected quarter: the Palace itself.

Queen Victoria had been interested in chloroform almost from the beginning, as evidenced by letters to her friend and closest confidante, the Duchess of Sutherland:

Windsor Castle, 11/16/49. My dearest duchess, ... your accounts of the chloroform are very interesting. The mode of giving it in a small dose and with so good an effect and yet without that loss of consciousness sounds most satisfactory ... Was Evelyn unconscious and did she inhale it or take it?

Osborne, 12/15/49. My dear duchess, I have to thank you for a kind letter with Dr Simpson's curious & interesting pamphlet. I have just had an opportunity of hearing from Lady Normamby the details of Lady Harwicke's confinement who used the chloroform & writes how it has succeeded so *wonderfully* – relieving her of *all* suffering at the time, and also afterwards. How wonderful it is!

The Queen was in fact expecting her seventh child, Prince Arthur, at the time, but apparently either she or her doctors decided against chloroform for his birth in May 1850. Three years later Victoria, by then aged 33 and a seasoned pro in matters of childbirth, caused her physician, Sir James Clark, to call in Dr John Snow, an anaesthetist from Edinburgh and a colleague and supporter of Dr Simpson, to administer chloroform for the birth of her eighth.

In his diary entry for April 7, 1853, Dr Snow described the procedure: 'I commenced to give a little chloroform with each pain, by pouring about fifteen *minims* by measure in a folded handkerchief.'*

He went on to tell of the successful outcome: 'The infant was

---

* The handkerchief method of administering blessed chloroform persisted well into the twentieth century. My sister Nancy, born in 1904, had an abscessed toe when she was two years old. The doctor came, put a chloroformed handkerchief on her face, and started to lance the toe – when my father, present at all operations to supervise the proceedings, saw that Nancy had stopped breathing. What did you do? we asked later. 'I seized the doctor by the neck and shook him.' Nancy survived; the fate of the hapless doctor is not recorded.

When I was about eight or nine (between 1925 and 1927) I had in rapid succession two broken arms – my proud boast, Two Arms Broken Before Ten. Each time, Dr Cheatle of Burford came to set the arm, and gave chloroform via the hankie method. 'Breathe deeply; you'll soon be asleep.' I can still remember the rather blissful feeling, odd concentric circles in one's closed eyes and waking up for a nice cup of tea.

When I was thirteen (1930), I had appendicitis – self-diagnosed, horrid pain in my stomach. I rang Dr Cheatle, who came over and took the appendix out, giving chloroform via hankie. Needless to say, all these procedures were done at home; none of us ever went to the hospital.

born at thirteen minutes past one by the clock in the room ...
consequently the chloroform was inhaled for fifty-three minutes.
The placenta was expelled in a very few minutes, and the Queen
appeared very cheerful and well, expressing herself much gratified
with the effect of the chloroform.'

For her part, the Queen was ecstatic. 'Dr Snow,' she wrote, 'gave
that blessed Chloroform & the effect was soothing, quieting &
delightful beyond measure.' This benediction from the Defender of
the Faith (a title held by all British monarchs) had a distinctly soothing and quieting effect on the clergy, further enhanced when a few
months later Dr Snow was called to Lambeth Palace, where he gave
chloroform to the Archbishop of Canterbury's daughter during her
accouchement. Thereafter, 'anaesthésie à la Reine' became all the
rage for those who could afford it.

Chloroform soon crossed the Atlantic, but was far less widely used
in America for childbirth than in England – possibly because for the
newly liberated Yankees high praise from the Queen of England
had less significance than for her country-women. The influential
Philadelphia physician Charles Meigs came out foursquare against
chloroform, declaring that 'There is, in natural labour, no element
of disease ... I should feel disposed to clothe me in sackcloth, and
cast ashes on my head for the remainder of my days, [if a patient
were to die from such] meddlesome midwifery.' (This is, incidentally,
the same Dr Meigs who came out foursquare against Dr Oliver
Wendell Holmes on the issue of causes of childbed fever.)

Actually, quite a few did die, enough to cause the Royal Medical
and Chirurgical Society of London to appoint a committee in 1863
to study the physiological effects of chloroform. By that time 123
deaths had been attributed to chloroform. Dr Simpson, ever ready
with a defence, pointed out that every year people are killed in train
accidents, or drowned swimming – would trains, then, be abolished?
And the healthful practice of sea bathing outlawed?

The centuries following the Chamberlens' invention of forceps saw
an explosion of scientific knowledge of human anatomy and its mysterious workings. Yet it was not until the late 1880s, three hundred
years post-Chamberlen, that the next great technological advance in

treating women endangered by unusually difficult labour was applied: delivery by Caesarean.

As every schoolchild knows, the term Caesarean derives from the birth of Julius Caesar, who was cut out of his mother's womb. Even the *Encyclopedia Britannica* gives half-hearted credence to this view in its definition: 'The operation for removal of a foetus from the uterus by an abdominal incision, so called from a legend of its employment at the birth of Julius Caesar.' However, spoilsport pedants point out that since Caesar's mother survived, in an era long before development of techniques to preserve the lives of both mother and baby, this must be incorrect. The true derivation, they insist, is from the Latin *caesura*, a cutting.

Be that as it may, the practice of cutting into dead or moribund mothers to preserve, if possible, a live infant is many centuries old. In Ancient Rome the law required that every woman dying in advanced pregnancy should be so treated; likewise in 1608 the Senate of Venice made it a criminal offence for any practitioner to fail to perform this operation on a pregnant woman thought to be dead.

The first known Caesarean birth in which both mother and child survived was achieved by Jacob Nufer, a Swiss pig-gelder, who in the year 1500 put his handy gelding tools to good use, operating on his wife after the doctors had given her up. Not only did Frau Nufer and her baby come through the ordeal, but she went on to have four more children by normal vaginal birth, thus disproving the twentieth-century medical dogma 'once a Caesarean, always a Caesarean'.

Over the next several centuries scattered reports surfaced from time to time of successful Caesareans that saved the lives of both mother and child; but these are mostly discounted by medical scholars as insufficiently documented and probably apocryphal. Doctors were understandably reluctant to try a Caesarean because even if they could produce a live baby, the mother almost invariably succumbed to massive haemorrhage and/or blood poisoning.

The first modern version of the operation was performed by a German doctor, Max Sänger, in 1882, by which time the discoveries of Pasteur and Lister about the causes of infection and the use of antiseptic techniques were well known. Furthermore, anaesthetic was now available. Dr Sänger's ingenious innovation was suturing the uterine wall as well as the abdominal wall with silk threads, plus the use of aseptic methods. He operated mainly on women with deformed pelvises, making a twelve-inch vertical incision from which he extracted the baby feet first, followed by the placenta. He reported an amazing success rate of 80 per cent.

Eventually the good news crossed the Atlantic. In Boston, a Caesarean was for the first time successfully performed in 1894 on a small woman with a tiny pelvis who had previously lost two babies. An eyewitness, describing the uterus, which was lifted through the incision and placed on the mother's skin, was clearly fascinated: 'This enormous organ, the color of a ripe plum, was a sight that filled the eyes of the beholder with wonder and respect . . . [Dr] Haven sutured the uterus in the approved Sänger manner, using silk . . . and closed the abdomen in the same way.' Thereafter the Sänger operation became known as the 'classic Caesarean', of which the many subsequent improvements were offshoots.

By the end of the nineteenth century, the contour of things to come on the American birth scene was clearly prefigured. Medicine was now firmly established as a gentleman's profession, and obstetrics as a major sub-specialty of this honourable calling; the discoveries of Pasteur and Lister had largely laid to rest the fear of infection as a cause of maternal death; blessed chloroform had allayed the terror of unendurable agony; forceps, their design vastly improved over the ancient Chamberlen model, were routinely used by the trained obstetrician; and finally, in a triumphant burst of scientific knowhow, the Caesarean operation had become available in cases of extreme emergency to save the lives of mother and infant.

The age of technology had arrived. From the obstetrician's point of view, the ideal venue for a safe delivery was the hospital, where he would have at hand all the most modern tools and accoutrements, not to mention the convenience to him of having the labouring mothers all in one place where assembly-line efficiency could be practised.

Soon, private patients, those who could afford to pay a doctor's fee plus the cost of a hospital stay, began to patronise the hospital as an appropriate place to have their babies. At first a trickle, maternity patients became a torrent. In the year 1900, less than five per cent of all American births took place in hospitals; by 1939, 50 per cent of all women and 75 per cent of urban women chose hospitals for the purpose; by 1970, the figure had risen to close to 100 per cent.

PART TWO

Modern Times

Chapter 3

FASHIONS IN CHILDBIRTH

In childbirth, as in other human endeavours, fashions start with the rich, are then adopted by the aspirant middle class with an assist from the ever-watchful media, and may or may not eventually filter down to the poor.

Beginning in the early years of the twentieth century, more and more well-to-do American women chose hospitals as the site of their lying-in. This was much encouraged by the medical profession, for several reasons: it relieved the family doctor of long hours at the patient's bedside waiting for the birth to happen; it gave impetus to the development of obstetrics as a medical specialty; it allowed for bringing into play the ever-proliferating technological improvements that were only available in a hospital setting; and it mandated complete control of parturition by doctors to the exclusion of midwives, marking another step in the passing of power over the birth process from traditional female to professional male. (There has been something of a parallel development in England, except that there, the really rich never have adjusted to the idea of turning out of their commodious, well-staffed houses into the sterile and regimented atmosphere of a hospital. In the 1980s it was still a matter of surprise and comment when the Princess of Wales decided to have her first-born in a hospital.)

For the expectant mother, an overriding consideration in choice of hospital over home birth was the promise held out by the former of alleviation of pain, via ever-more up-to-date anaesthetics for those who could afford them.

Looking over the literature on pain in childbirth, beginning with the Bible (as God said to Eve in one of His bad moods, 'In sorrow shalt thou bring forth children'), one can readily appreciate the terror that assailed women at the prospect. Actually God's injunction to Eve was mild compared to the horrendous description in the Church of England's *Book of Common Prayer* for 'The Thanksgiving of Women After Child-Birth': 'The snares of death compassed me round about; and the pains of hell gat hold upon me.' As a small child, wishing – like most children – to know precisely what was in store for me when I grew up, I remember reading and rereading this awful warning each Sunday morning in church, while the clergyman droned on with his dull sermon. My mother, asked what it felt like to have a baby, was hardly reassuring: 'Like an orange being stuffed up your nostril,' she said.

In view of these dire predictions, it's little wonder that a principal factor determining fashions in childbirth involved the whole matter of avoidance of pain, initially centred on the quest for the best available anaesthetic.

Shortly before World War I, numerous rich American women made pilgrimages to Germany for their accouchements, there to savour the delights of a new discovery, 'Twilight Sleep'. Having partaken of this miracle, they couldn't praise it enough; not only was delivery completely painless, they said, but their babies turned out amazingly healthy, beautiful, and intelligent. Arbiters of fashion, society leaders like Mrs John Jacob Astor, joined forces with feminists in a campaign to end once and for all the scourge of suffering in childbirth. Newspapers and magazines took up the cause. In 1915, the Twilight Sleep Maternity Hospital was established in Boston under the leadership of Dr Eliza Taylor Ransom, founder of the New England Twilight Sleep Association.

Confronted by this deluge of influential female demand, doctors and hospitals soon fell into line, and by the late 1930s Twilight Sleep had become the anaesthetic of choice, routinely administered in the more go-ahead hospitals along the Eastern seaboard. Obstetricians welcomed it because it gave them more control over the labouring woman than the chloroform/ether routine. Furthermore, the procedure resulted in an influx of paying patients, for whom the hospitals provided luxurious, tastefully decorated private wards, far from the cluttered institutional quarters of the charity patients.

The ingredients that produced the miracle of Twilight Sleep are akin to those used in the 'truth serum' we read about in sensational accounts of interrogations of prisoners of war and other captives at the mercy of their jailers. In 1940, Dr Joseph B. De Lee described the procedure as applied to the captive patient at the mercy of her obstetrician. 'Naturally,' he wrote, 'the profession eagerly grasped this opportunity to relieve women of the pain of childbirth, and these drugs soon were extensively employed here and abroad.'

In Twilight Sleep, hypodermic injections of morphine combined with scopalomine (a powerful hallucinogenic and amnesiac) and pentobarbital sodium were given every hour:

> The object is to maintain the patient in a state of amnesia, and this is determined by testing her memory ... Shortly after the second injection, the patient is asked if she remembers what has gone before, has she seen the nurse or intern? If she remembers, another dose is given. If not, nothing is done for an hour, when, if the mind seems to be clearer, 1/300 grain of scopalomine is given. Care must be exercised that the woman does not attain full consciousness ...
>
> During the pains she moves about restlessly, or turns from one side to the other, or grunts a little, and occasionally opens her eyes. She will respond to questions, but incoherently. As the second stage [movement of the baby out of the cervix into the birth canal] draws near its end she bears down and becomes very restless. Occasionally this becomes extreme, and several nurses are required to hold her ... A few whiffs of ether are often needed as the head passes through the vulva.

A graphic description of Twilight Sleep as witnessed by a father appeared in *They All Hold Swords*, a memoir of pre-World War II days by Cedric Belfrage. Cedric and his wife, Molly Castle, both young, adventurous British journalists, somehow ended up in Southern California for the birth of their baby in 1936. Thinking it would surely be a boy, they named the unborn child Fred. They chose a small bungalow hospital, a unique feature of which was that

Cedric was allowed to be present throughout the entire procedure – unheard of in those days.

The doctor explained that he would be giving Molly the first of several dopes which would blot out her memory. 'Soon, she began to moan ... Between two pains she said, "I hope you don't mind me crying out a bit now, darling. I could control my will before but now after the drugs I can't control it anymore."' As hours went by the doctor called the nurse to administer more injections. '"She will continue to show apparent signs of consciousness during the pains," he said. "But tomorrow she won't remember anything about it."'

Later, Molly was wheeled into the delivery room, where the doctor strapped her on to a table.

> The nurse put the nose-cap over Molly's face and began sprinkling ether on it from a perforated can ... Suddenly Molly seemed to come alive; she fought out wildly. Three of us were holding her, but she managed to wrench a hand free to claw frantically at the cap over her nose. She opened her eyes wide and gave a shrill, terrified scream. It was nearly a quarter of an hour before she was completely quiet again. The doctor remained calm, washing his hands over and over again in the corner. He said it was the dope she had had before that made her react this way to ether. She would remember nothing about it afterwards.
>
> She was snoring now, her body limp, her face almost covered by the ether cap. The doctor began probing with his great forceps. A lot of blood came ...
>
> He grasped something between the long, invisible arms of the forceps. He pulled hard ... He took a pair of scissors in one hand and in a careful, matter-of-fact way cut a slit to make the opening wider. A minute later the round object was almost out ... Everything was a mass of blood and I thought Fred must be dead already.

To Cedric Belfrage's untrained eye the newborn 'was exactly, in color and texture and size, like a large rabbit freshly skinned ... I could see that Fred was a girl.' The doctor slapped her; she yelped. Some hours later, when Molly woke up, 'I told her she had had a fine rabbit. She remembered nothing since the second shot in the arm, she said, except a vague nightmare memory of seeing people in gas-masks leaning over her, which made her think the war had started.'

So much for a father's viewpoint. Some observations by health professionals, beginning with Sheila Kitzinger, author of *The Complete Book of Pregnancy and Childbirth*:

> Many women have described it as 'twilight nightmare' because of its side effects. The usual amnesiac scopalomine (also known as 'scope' or 'the bomb') can cause total disorientation which may not end when the labour ends, thus its nightmarish quality. It is supposed to make women forget their labour but, in fact, most women report hazy memories of having felt like an animal howling in pain.

It was my impression from my own birth experiences in California, and those of various friends whose babies were born after 1940, that Twilight Sleep had vanished from the scene around the outbreak of World War II – presumably because of the potential dangers to mother and child of the massive amounts of anaesthetic required.

I was surprised to learn that this was not so. For decades after it was forsaken by the cognoscenti, Twilight Sleep was still used in out-of-the-way places, mainly for clinic patients, indigents or the uninsured.

In 1989 Dr Arlan Cohn, an internist in Berkeley, California, told me about 'a form of outrageous anaesthesia used at times during labour in the mid-fifties when I took my internship in St Louis. The mixture of scopalomine and Demerol or morphine injected into the mother resulted in an acute psychotic reaction during which the mother would scream out the darkest secrets of her life in a stream-of-consciousness babble that would have made James Joyce blush. The mother would then awake from this nightmare with total amnesia for her wild behaviour. God only knows what this crazy injection did to the foetal brain.'

Mary Welcome, a certified nurse-midwife practising in Atlanta, saw Twilight Sleep administered as late as 1974, when she was doing her nurse's training. In 1989 she told me, 'I can recall we would have hordes of labouring women – the doctors would knock them out, you know, with scopalomine, an amnesia drug, heavy-duty narcotics and sedatives. The women would be thrashing about in bed and yelling – but totally unaware of any of this. You had to put the rails up to keep them safe. Our nursing instructors told us you should be listening to the heartbeat every fifteen minutes, but the nurses would do this maybe twice in an eight-hour shift. And you'd look at their nursing records and realise that those women were left alone in there for hours. They were drugged up and knocked out. And the babies were often born unconscious themselves. You'd have to give them drugs to reverse the narcotics the mother had, and they'd stay sleepy for days.'

In 1990, in a belated effort to discover the precise nature of the anaesthetic I had endured in 1941 (hot air pumped up the rectum, as described on page 13 of Chapter 1), I consulted numerous local physicians, but none of them had ever heard of such a thing. They tactfully suggested that I might have been hallucinating after the inhalation of gas. One wrote, 'I'll bet my career that it was inhaled gas and not an enema that put you under. Gas anesthesia tends to scramble the mind of mother (and newborn) temporarily.' He added that the use of inhaled gas is now 'uniformly recognized as potentially very dangerous to mother and newborn.'

Eventually the mystery was solved, again by a passage from Joseph De Lee's *The Principles and Practice of Obstetrics*. He set forth the formula for 'rectal ether instillation' followed by a soothingly sophomoric lullaby presumably meant to be memorised by the attending obstetrician:

Early in the labor the patient is addressed as follows: 'Mrs —— , we are desirous of making your labor as painless as possible, and are prepared to do so without danger to you or your baby. Our success in relieving you will depend somewhat upon your cooperation. Therefore, when your pains become uncomfortable let the nurse know and she will give you two, or perhaps three, capsules (pentobarbital sodium, each 1½ grains) to relieve you.

'When your pains again become uncomfortable notify her as before and she will give you another capsule or two (pentobarbital sodium), or maybe a hypodermic (morphine sulfate, ⅙ or ¼ grain).

'Later, when this medicine begins to lose its effect, let her know and she will inject a solution into your rectum (ether-oil or ether-paraldehyde oil).'

Dr De Lee was an articulate and extremely influential early proponent of the notion that *all* births, including those designated 'low-risk', are inherently pathogenic and should be treated as such. 'It always strikes physicians as well as laymen as bizarre,' he wrote, 'to call labor an abnormal function, a disease, and yet it is a decidedly pathological process.'

His theories were sprung upon a waiting world – of obstetricians, that is – in his exhaustive *Principles and Practice*, a 1,200-page tome first published in 1913 and thereafter reprinted many times until 1940. A sampling of the De Lee philosophy, following his description of scientific advances in obstetrics:

This knowledge will raise the level and the dignity of our profession. Why is this process so slow? I believe, because, up to within a few years, the profession, and the public, considered childbirth to be a normal function, one requiring little medical supervision and hardly worth the attention of an expert surgeon . . .

It must be evident to anyone who will give the matter unbiased thought that, if we can invest obstetrics with the dignity of a great science, which it deserves, if we will acknowledge the pathogenic nature of this function, improvement will follow in every field of practice, and that anachronism, the midwife, will spontaneously disappear.

These concepts, incorporating as they did the twin aspirations of enhanced professional prestige and assured monopoly of their chosen field, were quickly embraced by De Lee's fellow practitioners. The fourfold remedy for the disease of childbirth, adapted from De Lee's teachings, continued to be standard practice in obstetrical wards for at least two generations. These were to be uniformly applied to *all* births, without distinction – forget about high risk/low risk. To summarise:

1. The patient should be placed in the 'lithotomy position'. (Incidentally, this expression was one I had not heard until I started

consorting with childbirth professionals, who told me it means
lying supine with legs in air, bent and wide apart, supported
by stirrups. However, the *Oxford English Dictionary* gives but
one definition: 'Lithotomy: The operation or art of cutting
for stone in the bladder'.)

2. She should be sedated from the first stage of labour.
3. The physician should perform an episiotomy, a cut of several
   inches through the skin and muscles between the vagina and
   anus to enlarge the space through which the baby must pass.
4. The physician should use forceps to effectuate delivery.

These measures, De Lee emphasised, could offset the dangers of
unaided birth, in which 'only a small minority of women escape
damage by the direct action of the natural process itself. So frequent
are these bad effects, that I have often wondered whether Nature
did not deliberately intend women to be used up in the process of
reproduction, in a manner analogous to that of the salmon, which
dies after spawning.'

The opening shot in defence of the spawning salmon, heretofore
voiceless sufferers caught in a net of obstetrical procedures, came
from a most unlikely quarter: *The Ladies' Home Journal*, which in
1957 and 1958 ran a series of hair-raising letters on the subject.

To put this in context: The *LHJ* was then, is now, and ever shall be
one of those multimillion-circulation women's mags whose essential
loyalty is to their advertisers, their contents generally consisting of
short, exhortative text pieces on how to be a better wife/mother, how
to dress better for less, how to cook for a crowd of teenagers, etc.,
surrounded by lovely huge colour ads bearing approximately the
same message. In *The Feminine Mystique*, published in 1963, Betty
Friedan plunged into a devastating analysis and critique of the insipid
outpourings of these magazines, one of her examples being the *LHJ*.
Combing through issue after issue of the late 1950s, she turned up
some marvellous plums for her chapter titled 'The Happy Housewife
Heroine'. Yet buried somewhere in those issues was a remarkable
correspondence starkly headlined 'Cruelty in the Maternity Wards'.

Why – and how – the ultra-respectable, superbland *LHJ* got
involved in a head-on confrontation with the American medical

establishment remains a mystery. In 1990, I wrote to the present editor asking for enlightenment; she did not answer my letter. I can only conclude that it was one of those unpredictable moments in the life of a nation, an individual, or in this case a magazine, when a steamroller of pent-up anger may have overridden normal editorial caution.

In any event, in November 1957 *The Ladies' Home Journal* published a brief letter in its reader-mail column from a registered nurse (name withheld at her request, as she feared reprisals from the medical community) asking for an investigation of 'the tortures that go on in modern delivery rooms':

> I have seen doctors who have charming examination-room manners show traces of sadism in the delivery room. One I know does cutting and suturing without anesthetic. He has nurses use a mask to stifle the patient's outcry.

> Great strides have been made in maternal care, but some doctors still say, 'Tie them down so they won't give us any trouble.'

Six months later, the *LHJ* editor reported a flood of letters relating childbirth experiences 'so shocking that they deserve national attention'. The May 1958 issue devoted many pages to excerpts from this outpouring of complaints, adding the requisite sententious disclaimer that 'the *Journal* does not question that the overwhelming majority of obstetricians and maternity hospitals resent such practices'.

A few quotations from the *LHJ*'s letters to the editor of May 1958 convey the general feeling. A mother of three, all born in different hospitals with different doctors, seemed dismayed at the yawning chasm between promise and reality:

> The practice of obstetrics is the most modern and medieval, the kindest to mothers and the cruelest. I know of many instances of cruelty, stupidity and harm done to mothers by obstetricians who are callous or completely indifferent . . . Women are herded like sheep through an obstetrical assembly line, are drugged and strapped on tables while their babies are forceps-delivered. Obstetricians today are businessmen who run baby factories.

Another wrote:

I was immediately rushed into the labor room. A nurse prepared me. Then, with leather cuffs strapped around my wrists and legs, I was left alone for nearly eight hours, until the actual delivery.

Recurrent complaints concerned the strapping down of the labouring mother; the prohibition of the father's presence during labour and delivery; and the general assembly-line atmosphere.

The May issue gave rise to yet another avalanche of letters, many of which were printed in the issue of December 1958:

Far too many doctors, nurses and hospitals seem to assume that just because a woman is about to give birth she becomes a nitwit, an incompetent, reduced to the status of a cow (and not too valuable a cow, at that) . . .

I was strapped to the delivery table on Saturday morning and lay there until I was delivered on Sunday afternoon. When I slipped my hand from the strap to wipe sweat from my face I was severely reprimanded by the nurse . . . For thirty-six hours my husband didn't know whether I was living or dead. I would have given anything if I could just have held his hand.

Some reported babies born dead, or hopelessly brain-damaged, victims (the writers suspected) of obstetrician-mandated delayed delivery and too much anaesthetic.

With few exceptions, the doctors who responded to these allegations against the profession issued blanket denials; nothing of the kind ever happened in *their* hospitals. An obstetrician's wife wrote indignantly of the many sacrifices she had made: 'I have broken many an engagement, kept many dinners warm, and cut vacations short because of my husband's concern for his patients.' Well, really! Aren't these minor inconveniences supposed to be a normal part of any conscientious doctor's way of life?

Nurses, also, had their say. Like the registered nurse whose letter originally stirred up the hornet's nest, these asked for protective anonymity. Most came down squarely on the side of the complaining mothers, and deplored the mentality of the profession:

Because of what is politely termed 'medical ethics', the truth of much bad practice is kept from the public. Personally I feel it is comparable to the 'ethics' which keeps criminals from telling on their accomplices ... What makes me angry is that the incompetent and unscrupulous people get away with so much.

Whether or not these *cris de coeur* had any direct effect on the development of a feminist birth philosophy as a feature of the women's liberation movement, then some years in the future, is at this late stage a matter of conjecture.*

In any event, predating the women's movement of the sixties and seventies, there arose a new phenomenon: 'natural childbirth', originating with the 1933 publication of *Natural Childbirth* (later called *Childbirth Without Fear*) by an English obstetrician, Dr Grantly Dick-Read. This was superseded in the 1950s by the work of Dr Fernand Lamaze, a French physician whose methods derived from Pavlovian theories he had studied in the Soviet Union. Thus, as in the case of Twilight Sleep, the innovators were foreign male physicians, and the first Americans to explore the possibilities offered by the new techniques were well-to-do women who travelled to Europe for the purpose.

On the face of it, the two systems seem similar. Dr Dick-Read's view was that the pains of childbirth are largely caused by fear-induced tension, which could be greatly ameliorated by instruction ahead of time about the childbearing process combined with classes in relaxation, exercises to keep the body supple, and training in deep breathing. Lamaze's method, which he called '*accouchement sans douleur*' (labour without pain), also required prenatal instruction in the physiology of pregnancy and labour, limbering-up exercises and breathing techniques – he favoured rapid, shallow panting over Dr Dick-Read's deep breathing.

Be that as it may – whether one is a deep breather or a shallow panter – the medical establishment after some initial resistance adopted (and modified for its convenience) the concept of natural childbirth and its concomitant, prenatal classes in which a lecturer trained in the method explains how it's done. Beginning in the 1970s

---

* *The Ladies' Home Journal* series is, however, mentioned in several of the books I consulted, including Wertz and Wertz's *Lying-In*, Margot Edwards and Mary Waldorf's *Reclaiming Birth*.

as a response to the women's movement, these classes are now routinely offered in the posher US hospitals under the umbrella term
'prepared childbirth'. Fathers, married or unmarried (discreetly
termed 'partners' in the promotional lit), are cordially invited to
come and breathe along in class, and if inclined are welcome to stay
in the hospital throughout the labour and delivery.

(Incidentally, the 'prepared childbirth' sessions are not to be con-
fused with prenatal care, in which from the earliest stages of pregnancy the expectant mother goes for regularly scheduled visits to her
midwife or to her obstetrician for physical examination, advice on
nutrition, and the ubiquitous tests of urine, blood, etc. Prenatal care
is universally thought to be an essential preamble to a successful
outcome: midwives, obstetricians, experts here and abroad, are
united in its advocacy.)

Also-rans in the natural-birth sweeps – but nevertheless influential
voices – were Robert Bradley of Denver and a French physician,
Frédérick Leboyer. While each had his share of enthusiastic supporters, both to some extent eventually fell afoul of the feminist
movement.

Dr Bradley, a pioneer of 'husband-coached childbirth' (the title of
his book published in 1965 by Harper & Row), was implacably
opposed to the use of drugs in childbirth, and himself presided over
some thirteen thousand drug-free births in which the husband-coach
was a full participant. But he used unfortunate terminology, referring
to the uterus as the 'baby box' and the clitoris as the 'passion button'.
It seemed to some women that Bradley was enlisting husbands in a
male power alliance in which husband and obstetrician became the
benign custodians of the little woman's physiology and behaviour.
Bradley's reputation was not enhanced when he remarked to a father,
'Let's face a fact: they [pregnant women] are nuttier than a fruitcake.'

Unlike others of his contemporaries – Lamaze, Dick-Read, Bradley, et al, – who had embraced the cause of natural childbirth,
Leboyer had scant sympathy for the labouring mother. On the contrary, his pity was all for the struggling foetus trying desperately to
make its way through the rigid birth canal into an alien environment.

To help it recover from this horrible experience, he advocated 'gentle birth', described in his book *Birth Without Violence* (New York: Knopf, 1975). The delivery room should be dimly lit and all present very quiet – Leboyer didn't much like having fathers around, as they are apt to exclaim loudly at the first sight of the newborn. As soon as the babe emerged, Leboyer lowered it into a lukewarm bath, simulating its former watery home. For a soft and kindly introduction to its fellow human beings, Leboyer – *not* the mother – would give the baby a gentle, reassuring massage; only then would the mother be given it to hold.

As for the mother, Leboyer surmised that for the baby she must appear to be a monster incarnate. At the onset of labour it finds itself being crushed, stifled, assaulted:

> With its heart bursting, the infant sinks into hell ... the mother is driving it out. At the same time she is holding it in, preventing its passage. It is she who is the enemy. She who stands between the child and life. Only one of them can prevail. It is mortal combat ... not satisfied with crushing, the monster twists it in a refinement of cruelty.

Women who welcome Leboyer's advocacy of softly lit, quiet labour rooms in contrast to the bright lights and constant banging about encountered in many hospitals – and may also favour a nice warm bath for the newborn – can hardly be expected to choke down the rest of his strangely misogynistic views of motherhood.

The dramatic transformation of the father's role from the 1960s to the late 1980s is described by Warren Hinckle III, who sampled both. Hink Three, as I call him for short, was one of the trio of *Ramparts* editors, all under thirty, who in the 1960s tweaked the noses of President Johnson, the CIA, and the military with stunning exposés that contributed in no small measure to LBJ's downfall and the eventual ending of the Vietnam War. 'Never trust anybody over thirty!' was the slogan of Hink Three and his editorial colleagues, Robert Scheer and Dugald Stermer.

Hinckle's account of fatherhood in the sixties:

> In Irish San Francisco, birthing was a simple division of labor: The woman went to the hospital, and the man went to the bar.

The intimate details of birth were left to the mother and the mother-in-law on the reasonable ground that they had experience in such matters.

I waited for the birth of my first two children in the yellow half-light of Cookie Picetti's Star Cafe on Kearny Street. They were born three years apart but the theater of nativity remained the same: The phone rang in the bar. Cookie picked up the receiver and listened intently. A smile as broad as a barge crossed his face. 'Ya godda goil,' said Cookie. He hung up the phone. I bought drinks for the house. The house bought drinks back.

Onward to 1989. The goils are grown up and Warren Hinckle is remarried, his wife, Susan Cheever, expecting some time in November. They are living in New York; although Hink Three is now in his fifties, his description of the Blessed Event seems perfectly trustworthy:

On the night of the earthquake [October 17, 1989] I was dragooned in a Lamaze class on the fifth floor of a grotty office building on New York's upper East Side, seated next to a Dentyne-popping yuppie.

'Now, everyone take off their shoes and get on the floor and the men can practice being human labor tables,' said the instructor. She had a computer voice with a programmed smile.

When the men had been human labor tables long enough, there was a lot of huff-and-puff practice pain control breathing – 'Let's take a deep, cleansing breath,' said the computer voice. I excused myself to go to the bathroom and raced downstairs to a bar across the street and watched San Francisco burn on the television.

Back upstairs at the pain factory the ladies had finished breathing and the men were putting their penny loafers back on and there was the smell of socks in the air.

'Now you guys just remember that you're glued in the labor room with your partner – you can't move an inch, you can wait to pee until after the baby is born,' the instructor said, giggling girlishly.

A couple of weeks later, the scene shifts to Mount Sinai hospital, where Dr Herbert Jaffin decides to try for vaginal delivery, although Susan, aged forty-six, had had a previous Caesarean. Jaffin recommends the posture of '*Sitzfleisch*, loosely translated as sitting on your butt'. Later, he proceeds 'to violate the scripture of the more puritanical "natural birth" advocates' by administering Pitocin and an epidural.

At the moment of birth, Dr Jaffin 'waved his tools [forceps] like a matador and proceeded to his art.

'Suddenly the baby was there all red, white and blue – blue of skin and red with blood and the goop of birth, with the whites of his eyes flashing, arms waving and flapping in the air.'

Thus the triumphal entry of Warren Hinckle IV, also known by me as Hink Four but called Quad by his proud parents and their friends; clearly an occasion of exhilaration for his doting papa.

Autre temps, autres moeurs. John Kenneth Galbraith in June 1989, answering a letter in which I had mentioned that I was writing this book, observed:

Alas, it is a subject to which I had not previously given more than three minutes' thought. Kitty and I had, over the years, discussed the circumstances which caused her, while in perfect health, to be confined to the hospital for a full 10 days when Alan was born, now close on to 50 years ago. Our offspring handled the whole situation in approximately two days. Anyhow, quite clearly this is something to be explored.

Yes, but also worth exploring is Professor Galbraith's not previously having given more than three minutes' thought to the subject. This conjures up the picture of his wife, Kitty, struggling bravely, solo, with the pangs of labour while JKG, busy man that he always was (and is), occupies himself with vital problems of national and international import.

If the scene could be re-enacted today, we might visualise Galbraith being dragged by a giant hook, like those used in French theatres to remove unpopular performers, off the world stage and into his wife's delivery chamber. There his attention would be concentrated for a lot more than three minutes, as he breathes and strains, à la Dick-Read or Lamaze, in unison with Kitty until the great moment when he is called upon to himself cut the umbilical cord.

In the wake of these developments, new inventions mushroomed, some eminently sensible, others wild enough to qualify for Ripley's *Believe It Or Not*.

Item: Birthing stool, advertised in Ina May Gaskin's quarterly publication *The Birth Gazette*. The stool is adapted from that used by centuries of midwives, whose kit included a wooden contraption that looks something like a toilet seat (minus, obviously, a watery flush), for squatting on during labour. The modern version is (according to the ad) 'finely handcrafted of pine, leather and 4″ foam', and looks quite comfy for the purpose.

Item: Another *sitzfleisch* gadget, the birth cushion, invented by Jason Gardosi of St Mary's Hospital in London. Like the birthing stool, it is designed to support the thighs and allow for squatting deliveries. According to the London *Independent*, this method had 'almost halved forceps deliveries of first babies, shortened second stage labour and resulted in less injury to the mother'. At least sixty National Health Service hospitals were offering British maternity patients the option of using the cushion.

Item: Underwater birth. I went to see a documentary film on this called *Water Baby*, produced and introduced by Karil Daniels of Point of View Productions. The movie shows practitioners delivering babies underwater in three countries: in the Soviet Union, Igor Charkovsky, who first promulgated the idea in the 1960s ('He's not a doctor, he's a boat builder', I was told by Sheila Kitzinger, who is something less than a fan); in France, Dr Michel Odent of the Centre Hospitalier Général de Pithiviers, who in *The Lancet* of December 24, 1983, reported the 100th birth under water in his hospital, almost all without subsequent complications; and in the United States, Dr Michael Rosenthal, obstetrician of the Family Birthing Center in Upland, California.

Underwater labour, viz., lying in a warm bath to ease the discomfort of contractions in the early stages, allowing as it does for freedom of movement without the pull of gravity, has long been an option offered by midwives and other home-birth advocates. But in *Water Baby* we see the infant's head, body, and legs slowly emerging in a small birthing pool, sometimes with the enthusiastic 'partner' alongside the mom. Having been accustomed to a watery environment for nine months, the commentator explains, the babe rather likes this. It doesn't need to breathe until the cord is cut, as it still gets oxygen from that source.

'Do many babies drown?' I asked nervously. Hardly any, Karil Daniels said; she had heard of only one case, rumoured but never authenticated, in which the parents did it all by themselves in the family bathtub without a trained birth attendant.

Rather to my surprise – and relief – Ina May Gaskin, that birth innovator *par excellence* (about whom more in Chapter 12), voiced the same misgivings. She didn't know how many documented cases of foetal deaths had been attributable to underwater births; but she did feel that two of the births shown in Karil Daniels's film 'came dangerously near the edge'. She also questioned the hygienic precautions, especially when other people – birth assistants and those ever-present 'partners' – plunge full of enthusiasm into the tub along with mom and the unborn babe.

Ms Gaskin's main, eminently commonsensical, observation is that since our ancestors from time immemorial were born into air, along with all other mammals – puppies, kittens, giraffes, elephants, etc. – why disturb the natural order?

Item: Heading into the Twilight Zone, we learn of the Empathy Belly, designed by Linda Ware, a 'prenatal educator' in Redmond, Washington. The belly, consisting of a huge womblike structure with large breasts, priced at $595, is designed to be worn by the male partner so that he can appreciate the discomfort of the later stages of pregnancy. It weighs thirty-five pounds, is guaranteed to cause backache, shortness of breath and fatigue, and comes with a special pouch that presses on the wearer's bladder, creating an uncomfortable desire to urinate at inappropriate moments. According to its inventor, 'a half hour in the Empathy Belly teaches a man more about what goes on during pregnancy. He ends up being more understanding and supportive about what a woman goes through. For most men, it opens up a new world of feelings. It's something they think about and enjoy.' In short, the perfect Father's Day gift for the likes of Hink Three or J. K. Galbraith.

Item: The Uterine University. In a development of the notion that one is never too young to learn, prenatal educators from Florida to Washington state are promoting devices for the *in utero* education of the foetus.

Offerings include Fetal Teaching Systems, cassettes to be worn by the mother-to-be on a body-belt, available from Mr Shannon Thomas of Orlando, Florida; the 'Listen Baby' fabric belt with two speakers and a little microphone, from Roger Hurst of Infant Technology in Denver; and the Pregaphone, invented by Dr Rene Van de Carr of Santa Barbara, California.

Whether the foetus, swimming about in its amniotic fluid, enjoys the lessons – or whether it is bored by the whole idea – has not yet been fully researched, although Dr Brent Logan of the Washington Institute of Prenatal Education in Snohomish does record a baby saying 'Gogo' three times shortly after delivery. 'The nurses were amazed,' he said. (The newborn's utterance is, it seems to me, subject to at least two interpretations: was it saying 'Go! Go!' meaning 'Leave me alone!' or simply burping like any illiterate?)

Item: In what must be one of the most imaginative lawsuits of recent years, attorney Michael Box filed suit in Jefferson City, Missouri, contending that the state is illegally imprisoning an inmate's foetus. Box cited Missouri's anti-abortion law, which says life begins at conception. If that is so, he said, 'then fetuses are supposed to be like anyone else – they're a person, and they have constitutional rights.'

He contends that key provisions of the Missouri law, upheld by the US Supreme Court in its July 1989 ruling on the abortion issue, extend to the unborn 'all the rights, privileges and immunities available to other persons'. Hence the foetus (whose mother-to-be is serving a three-year sentence for forgery and stealing) has been illegally imprisoned – having itself never been charged with a crime, allowed to consult an attorney, convicted, or sentenced.

If this legal theory should prevail, will the courts be bombarded with Writs of Habeas Foetus?

*

Aside from some of the zanier products of the ever-fertile American entrepreneurial imagination, there seems to be no doubt that for the affluent, and those with large, inclusive health insurance policies, hospital birth today can be a highly enjoyable experience.

Vying to capture the carriage trade, hospitals outdo each other in advertising birth *à la mode*, which, they assure us, offers all the cosy benefits of home birth in a safe hospital setting. Latching on to the popularity and publicity surrounding the home-birth movement of the 1970s, a typical ad like one from Eden Hospital in Castro Valley, California, shows a couple and baby with the headline 'Having My Baby at Eden Was So Comforting, Almost Like Delivering at Home.' At HCA West Paces Ferry Hospital in Atlanta, 'Birthing suites feature early American furniture complete with a four-poster bed and a charming cradle'. (Cost: $7,000 minimum.) Most offer rooming-in with the mother for the baby and the father, who – perhaps in deference to the shadow of Dr Semmelweis – is asked to wash his hands. Not only fathers, but siblings and anyone else the mother wants to invite are welcome to attend the birth. A champagne dinner for two served in the mother's room concludes this magnificent birthday treat.

In Alexandria, Virginia, in April 1990, I went to see the Alexandria Hospital, which, I was told, is the preferred place for yuppie births. This offers all the above-described advantages plus a pink dining room called 'Le Bébé' with fresh flowers on each table for two, where the new parents can choose among filet mignon, 'catch of the day' and chicken Kiev.

I can visualise a TV mini-series segment showing the delighted parents as they depart from these charming surroundings, clasping their pink bébé (there would be few of darker hue) and its brand-new Vuitton nappy carrier. In the final scene, they enter their comfortable dwelling, a bower of flowers sent by well-wishers, all to the background music of the Brahms Lullaby.

Chapter 4

THE IMPOVERISHED WAY

As the disgraceful statistics show year after year, the United States, with the highest per capita expenditure on health care of any country in the world, ranks twenty-fourth among Western industrial nations in infant mortality, due entirely to the not-so-benign political and bureaucratic neglect of the very poor, the uninsured (comprising an astonishing thirty-seven million Americans, in 1990, up from 28.6 million in 1980), teenage mothers, and those who are alcoholic or drug-addicted.

Focusing in for a close look at one example of the miserable experience confronting these women and their babies, a PBS crew directed by Robert Thurber produced a 1989 documentary called *Babies at Risk*, featuring Chicago's Cook County Hospital, where more than five thousand women were delivering babies each year. Some were on Medicaid, a national scheme for which the indigent are eligible, but a growing number had no insurance at all.

In this film, which as the producers have pointed out is merely illustrative of a situation that exists in every major US city, we are shown agonising pictures of skeletal newborns stuck full of tubes, struggling for life in their incubators. Thanks to modern technology, most could be expected to survive – but would be likely to require long periods of costly hospitalisation throughout life. For starters, each day in the neonatal intensive care unit when the documentary was made cost $1,200. The average stay was about twenty days, or $24,000 a baby.

As for prenatal care – which the doctors believed could have prevented many of these disastrous outcomes for the baby – it was virtually non-existent for their mothers. Since 1986, nine of Chicago's community hospitals serving poor communities had closed, due in large part to the growing number of uninsured patients and the low rate of reimbursement by Medicaid. Many of Chicago's better hospitals refused to accept poor women; instead, they transferred them to Cook County even if they were in advanced labour, a highly dangerous procedure known as 'dumping'.

According to the film, a pregnant woman seeking prenatal care in the clinics run by the Chicago Department of Health might have to wait as long as nine weeks before being given an appointment. Once this was accomplished, she might wait all day before she could see an obstetrician.

Gladly willing to fill this vacuum – and thereby bilk the taxpayer of a tidy sum – were private doctors who conduct a thriving business in storefront clinics in the poor Chicago neighbourhoods, where they hold out the promise of prenatal care to Medicaid patients. Known by Cook County health professionals as 'Medicaid mills', the clinics were charging Medicaid $28 per patient visit. They crammed in as many women as possible in any given day, doing virtually nothing for them – 'The person loses, the taxpayer loses, and it's the worst kind of ripoff,' said Jerry Stermer, president of Voices for Illinois Children. As Dr Linda Powell of Cook County Hospital pointed out, 'That's as bad, if not worse, than no prenatal care because the patients think they are having good care and they think everything's OK and in fact it's not, and they have very, very severe problems when they come to us.'

So why haven't these bad actors been run out of the medical profession? Essentially, it would seem, because the Illinois State Medical Society, like its counterpart the California Medical Association (with its Board of Medical Quality Assurance), prefers to look the other way when fellow physicians might be 'at risk' – never mind the risk to patients and their babies.*

---

* A state-by-state list of licensing boards, furnished by BMQA in 1988, listed under the general heading 'Illinois Department of Professional Regulation' the subheads 'Medical Licensing Board' and 'Medical Disciplinary Board', each with several locations in Illinois. None was mentioned by name in *Babies at Risk*.

Aside from segments showing the heroic efforts of dedicated public-health workers, swamped by the sheer volume of needy pregnant women, for this viewer the icing on the cake was provided by the Governor of Illinois, James Thompson, who explained on-camera:

Illinois has really been, since I've been governor, at the forefront of infant mortality initiatives. Our infant mortality ranking is skewed by the statistics from Chicago.

Well done, Governor. Worthy of one of those *New Yorker* filler items headed 'How's That Again?'

To get further specific details – the whys and wherefores, who is to blame, what if any solutions are in sight – I consulted Dr Barbara Allen, a black paediatrician who since 1981 has been director of maternal and child health for Alameda County, California. In this vast, mainly urban area with a highly diversified population including blacks, Hispanics, plus Asian immigrants, Dr Allen's job boggles the mind.

The great majority of her clientele are on Medi-Cal, the California medical assistance programme for families on welfare. Maternity facilities for these clients are in East Oakland at Highland, the county hospital, supplemented by eight public-health clinics scattered throughout the county where a woman can go for prenatal care. However, said Dr Allen, about 50 per cent of the women who do come in to Highland have had no prenatal care. Why? I asked. 'A variety of reasons. There's a hard-core group of women out there who are chemically dependent, whose addiction is so great that it's their primary reason for being, so prenatal care is not at all a priority in their minds. Some women out there are homeless and just walking from one place to another, and trying to get into prenatal care. Some try late in pregnancy to get care. And then a lot of clinics may not accept them late in pregnancy because by that time they are considered high-risk. Private doctors won't accept them late in pregnancy.'

What happens then? 'They either end up going to Highland emergency room or they just stay out of the system until it's time to deliver.' An increasing number deliver at home, Dr Allen told me – unattended, totally alone. 'Again, a lot of these women are chemically dependent, and in particular on crack cocaine. And some of them are just so isolated, disconnected. A larger and larger percentage of the mothers coming in are really destitute or chemically dependent or both.'

As to physicians in private practice, a tiny handful will accept Medi-Cal patients – and at that, they limit these to only two or three a month.

Infant mortality? 'The gap is widening,' Dr Allen said. 'In the non-black population the infant mortality rate and low-birth-weight rate continue to decline, but we see in the black population an increase in the rate.

'Anyway,' she said, 'infant mortality isn't really a medical issue. As long as our society has decided it's OK to have large numbers of people who have no place to live, just belong in the streets, who have insufficient food – no matter what the medical care, what we are finding is that they go right back into these dire living circumstances. So you may be telling her, "I want you to take this medication X amount of times a day," and if she's living on the streets somebody snatches her bag, her medication and so on.

'In order to correct the increase in infant mortality I think we're going to have to drastically modify how we see people in this society, especially the poor and the minorities in the community. It is always amazing to me when I hear what we're doing to fight drugs in other countries, the amount of money, and we're going to give them military technical assistance. Yet we have all these neighbourhoods that are suffering from drug epidemics and things are out of control, and we can't care, or we don't consider war on drugs right in our back-yards. It's like we've written off whole segments of our population.'

In Dr Allen's view, at least one answer would be a system 'where everybody can be assured access to health care, a well-thought-out national health insurance programme.' In other countries, she added, 'not only do they have that, but they have very good support programmes for women and families – mandatory maternity leave for employed mothers, extended paternity leave where they get extra stipends.'

Highland Hospital in East Oakland is a huge, forbidding, prison-like structure. Dr James Jackson, black chairman of the Department of Maternal and Child Health and Chief of Obstetrics, has worked there since 1984, when he quit his private practice at Alta Bates Hospital to work for the county.

It has been a period of phenomenal growth, he told me. Births at Highland sky-rocketed from fewer than 1,000 in 1981 to 2,800 in 1989. When Dr Jackson first came, he had two physicians in the obstetrics department; in 1989, he had eleven. An indispensable component is the group of twelve certified nurse-midwives, who 'do prenatal care on all of the normal patients and deliver more than half of the babies'.

Another huge change in the general obstetrical scene is the decline – almost to the vanishing point – of private doctors willing to take Medi-Cal patients. 'The worst thing a person can do is come into a doctor's office and wave a Medi-Cal card,' said Dr Jackson. 'You're like a pariah if you walk in with a Medi-Cal card. You can have a blue card, a green card, or any other card, but Medi-Cal has a bad reputation and connotation.'

So, what to do? Like Dr Allen, Dr Jackson thinks that 'medical intervention is to deal with illness, with poor outcomes. But we should be far more concerned with underlying causes. The social factors outweigh the medical factors.' Like Dr Allen, he supports a national, comprehensive health insurance law.

My introduction to the Alabama way of birth was a Pulitzer prize-winning series titled 'A Death in the Family' in the *Alabama Journal* of September 14 to 18, 1987, which gave the state's infant mortality rate (babies who die before the age of one year) as 13.3 per thousand live births, at a time when the national figure was 10.4. For black babies, the rate was 19.9, for white, 9.7, a ratio that holds true for most of the country.

The five-part series, replete with human-interest stories – heart-rending cases of grinding poverty and official dereliction – also afforded some glimpses into the politics of Alabama perinatal care for the indigent.

Governor Guy Hunt made rather good copy. Prodded by the reporters to explain his pocket veto of a legislative resolution calling

for expansion of Medicaid coverage, he took the Reaganesque forget-
tability route: 'I don't remember pocket-vetoing anything that dealt
with it.' His memory jogged by the persistent journalists, Hunt said
he probably vetoed it 'because it recommended that the amount
obstetricians are paid for a Medicaid delivery be increased from $450
to $750'.

Hunt disagreed with the opinion of some business experts that the
high infant mortality rate discourages companies from relocating to
Alabama because it indicates a poor quality of life. 'We have not
found this to be hindering our industrial development at the present
time,' he said, which has the ring of truth: corporations bent on
finding a cheap source of labour in a largely non-union state are
hardly likely to worry about the infant mortality rate amongst those
they seek to exploit.

The governor added, 'I think it should be pointed out that the
quality of care that we're receiving at a lot of our institutions in our
state is the highest of anywhere in the world,' a comment that
enraged public-health workers toiling in the front lines of the battle
to reduce infant mortality; for obvious reasons, they told the *Journal*
reporters, the poor are not recipients of the kind of care that Governor Hunt was talking about.

Even more infuriating was the governor's proposal for a task force
'to study the problem', that ever-handy device beloved by politicians
wishing to deflect the slings and arrows of outraged constituents. 'I
want to examine the issue thoroughly before committing funds,' he
told the reporters, to which an exasperated health consultant replied,
'We *know* about the problem. It shouldn't take long to study. You
don't have to reinvent the wheel.' And State Senator MacPherson:
'That means 600 more babies are going to die in the next year
without the attention they deserve. The problem has been studied
long enough.'

The cruellest blow of all was the *Journal*'s revelation that Mississippi, which in 1985 had held the distinction of being at the very
bottom of the fifty states in the infant death rate, had climbed to
eighth worst, leaving Alabama in the Number 50 spot. To put this
in context for readers unfamiliar with the particular sensitivities of
the states involved: Alabama and Mississippi tend to run neck and

neck in a perpetual race as to which is the worst in national statistics in just about anything to do with the public welfare: education, housing, mean annual income (and 'mean' is the *mot juste*), health care, sanitation, etc.

The *Journal*'s writing team donated its Pulitzer prize money to the Gift of Life Foundation, a newly organised Montgomery group 'dedicated to lowering the state's infant mortality rate'. In 1990, three years after the *Journal* series was published, I went to Montgomery to see Gift of Life in operation.

For starters, I met with Doris Barnette, acting director of the Alabama Department of Public Health's Family Health Service Bureau, whose functions include oversight of maternal and child care; the federal Special Supplemental Feeding Programme for Women, Infants, and Children (WIC); and family planning, among several other subtasks. Mrs Barnette is a large, expansive, charismatic woman who clearly inspires her staff and anyone else who comes into her orbit. As a staff member told me, 'She keeps us going by her sheer enthusiasm; just being around her is like a shot of adrenaline.' Mrs Barnette is a Southerner born and bred, originally from Louisiana, a social worker by training who spent some years in Mississippi in health work before coming to Alabama in 1986.

The Gift of Life programme, which functions under the aegis of her department, has accomplished a complete transformation in maternal care in Montgomery, she said: 'It's an example of what can be done when a community comes together. Due to Gift of Life Montgomery went from terrible to almost tolerable.'

As background, she described an audit done in 1987 by the General Accounting Office which 'found Montgomery was the worst place anywhere in the United States to have a baby. There were three hospitals where indigents could give birth. People without resources came to the health department to get prenatal care. The director was an old doctor, not sensitive at all to the needs of the patients. The clinics were overrun; patients averaged less than three prenatal visits, whereas the American College of Obstetricians and Gynecologists recommends thirteen visits for a normal pregnancy – and a large number of these were high-risk.'

Most nightmarish of all was the procedure for getting into a hospital once labour had started: 'The three hospitals that accepted indigents rotated what they called "Emergency Room of the Day". If you were pregnant and about to get ready to deliver, you had to listen to the radio at six a.m. to find out which was the E.R. of the day.'

Compounding the problems of women seeking prenatal care and admittance to a hospital for delivery was their wholesale abandonment by the medical profession. 'Ten years ago, four hundred fifty obstetricians and family-practice doctors were delivering babies,' said Mrs Barnette. 'Today it's less than two hundred, with practically no family physicians – less than twenty – delivering babies.' The reason: malpractice insurance premiums in Alabama have risen to an average of $50,000, up to $65,000 in some rural areas. Those 450 family doctors each used to deliver from thirty to forty babies annually out of a total of sixty thousand births in Alabama. When insurance companies forced them to pay premiums as high as those paid by obstetricians, they were forced to drop delivering babies from their practice. They couldn't even begin to pay the premiums with only thirty to forty deliveries per year.

'One of the fallouts from the malpractice situation is that doctors are refusing to take Medicaid patients because of their mistaken belief that poor people are more apt to sue for malpractice,' said Mrs Barnette. 'I don't believe this. There are no statistics to back it up – furthermore, in my experience, poor people in the rural areas are on the whole suspicious of lawyers, and are not likely to seek one out. You'll hear such comments as "When Uncle Joe was in trouble we got a lawyer and he charged plenty, but Joe went up to the penitentiary." But it's the perception of physicians that counts, and what keeps a lot of them from accepting Medicaid cases.'

In the four-county area surrounding Montgomery, Mrs Barnette told me, there had been some twenty-five doctors delivering babies in the early 1980s, but by 1987 there were only thirteen, and others were planning to get out. 'It was crisis. We were about to reach the point where every single obstetrician was about to stop delivering babies and you would not be able to have a baby in Montgomery or anywhere thereabouts, no matter what your income was.'

Into this horrible mess stepped the Gift of Life Foundation, through which obstetricians and certified nurse-midwives provide comprehensive prenatal care and counselling at county health department clinics serving Montgomery and surrounding rural areas. About eighteen hundred babies a year are delivered in two Montgomery hospitals, also under the auspices of Gift of Life. The clientele is 75 per cent black, 25 per cent white – there is no appreciable Hispanic population in the Montgomery area, Mrs Barnette said. In a typical year the programme will have three to five FTE, or full-time equivalent, physicians; one FTE may actually be two part-time doctors. Gift of Life has about eight certified nurse-midwives and is constantly looking for more, but CNMs are very hard to get. 'They're scarce as hens' teeth,' said Mrs Barnette. 'We are recruiting all we can find ... we hunt them, we hunt them.'

Like health professionals everywhere, Mrs Barnette is absolutely sold on the paramount importance of prenatal care in reducing the incidence of premature, low-weight births and ensuring a better outcome of the pregnancy. 'It's pure magic,' she said. 'We don't quite know what it is about prenatal care that makes it magic. We only know that more and better prenatal care results in better babies.'

Prenatal care as furnished by Gift of Life is a far cry from the crowded public-health clinic where a woman may wait for hours until she hears the words 'Next, please.' Ms Next, whether she is a seasoned mother of six or a terrified fourteen-year-old expecting her first, will typically get a perfunctory examination by somebody she has never seen before – and likely will never see again, as personnel are constantly rotated – and be speedily ejected to make way for the next Ms Next.

Not so in the Gift of Life set-up. As explained by Mrs Barnette and others in the programme, the goal is to arrange for each patient to be followed throughout her pregnancy by the same individual: 'This personal attention and concern may be the magic ingredient of prenatal care,' she said, and recited a poignant line from a poem to illustrate the point: '*I had a nurse who knew my name ...*'

A further step in the concept of maternity care as a one-on-one proposition is 'case management', a programme still in the initial stages as of 1990, designed to supplement the medical aspects of prenatal care. 'The pregnant woman,' said Mrs Barnette, 'is assigned *one* case manager, generally a social worker, to lead her by the hand through the highly confusing bureaucratic maze of services to which she is entitled. Where to get food stamps? How to apply for WIC benefits?

'What we have had are nurses who give the best prenatal care they can. But a nurse with a clinic and forty patients waiting to see her can't stop and, for example, help a single parent find housing. That's the sort of problem the case manager tries to cope with. An additional benefit is that the case manager is able to follow up the birth and see that the new mothers get into family-planning services for birth control. The object is to space the babies at least two years apart, but sometimes by the time a mother comes in for her postpartum check-up, she is pregnant again. That's because there was no one person working with them, before we started this programme.'

How much does all this cost and who pays for it? I asked. Needless to say, in a country whose proud and oft-repeated slogan is 'the bottom line is the dollar sign', this is a crucial question.

The budget for three physicians and eight certified nurse-midwives is $1.2 million a year, said Mrs Barnette. Start-up money for the Gift of Life Foundation came from a variety of sources, both public and private: the state health department, cities and counties, churches, some grant money, and (surprisingly) even gifts from almost a dozen doctors, to the tune of $1,000 each.

For further elucidation, Doris Barnette steered me to two other movers and shakers in the Gift of Life set-up: Dr John Porter, chairman of the foundation, whose idea it was in the first place, and Martha Jinright, director of the programme since its inception.

Before coming to Montgomery in 1981, Dr Porter served for some years (1976 to 1981) as the only obstetrician in a small town in Mississippi – population ten thousand, plus another twenty thousand in the surrounding rural areas. He seemed driven, like many another who ventures into the quagmire of maternity facilities for the indigent, by twin and complementary passions: a fervent desire to accomplish at the very least a decent professional standard of care for the patients, and an abiding hatred of obstructionist politicians and bureaucratic foot-draggers.

'The working poor don't qualify for Medicaid,' Dr Porter told me.

'Almost nobody in Alabama qualified. From 1981 to '87, I watched the horrendous time the poor had giving birth; there was not enough money from Medicaid and no private doctor would furnish prenatal care. The working poor and the indigent went to the health department for prenatal care but *not* for delivery. There was no continuity of care. Women just dropped into Emergency when they were already in labour. A bad system.'

At first, Dr Porter encountered nothing but discouragement in his campaign to improve the situation: 'We met with the county government, the county commissioners, the mayor, all the hospital administrators, and tried to get something accomplished. We got absolutely nowhere.

'The fact is the politicians are not interested in anything that won't get them votes. It's just not an issue that's important to them, because it was a bunch of poor people who didn't matter anyway.

'One day I got the idea, talking to my wife, that with more money from Medicaid plus private donations, we could hire CNMs and doctors.' Having enlisted the support of the health department and assorted paediatricians, Dr Porter and his colleagues raised enough money through private donations to employ four CNMs and two doctors. This proved to be an excellent goad with which to prod the politicians into action: 'I think we shamed them because the initial start-up money was all volunteer donations, from individuals and from churches.' Once the Gift of Life had proved to be outstandingly successful – and had across-the-board community support – the politicians soon swung behind it. 'A politician would be committing suicide if he tried to end this programme now,' said Porter. 'I think that you will find that the Gift of Life Foundation, how we did it and how we set it up, will be used as a prototype by many other communities.'

When the search began for a director of the Gift of Life project, there were over a hundred applicants. Martha Jinright, who had worked for some years with the March of Dimes, which seeks to prevent birth defects, was one of eight to make it to the final stage, an interview by a committee of community leaders charged with the final selection. As the programme was a brand-new proposition, the selection committee had little to go on, Ms Jinright told me. 'They called me back to tell me that I drew the short straw.'

She began working at the inauguration of the project, in May 1988. 'The Gift of Life started delivering in June of that year. We've delivered a little over three thousand in the twenty-two months that we've been in operation.'*

Martha Jinright identified the three factors which, she believes, contributed most to the success of Gift of Life: 'First, the nurse-midwives. I think we need our physicians – I don't want to short-change them, but I think we could have hired twenty physicians and not had the success we've had with the nurse-midwifery component. The hands-on, woman-to-woman relationship, the personal relation-ship is a real, vital part of the project.'

I was curious to know whether there was much opposition from Alabama physicians to the employment of nurse-midwives. 'Not from those in our programme,' said Ms Jinright. 'But yes – from several in the medical profession in general. I think we have – I don't know any other term to describe them – the old coots. You can't tell them anything. They see the midwives as a threat, taking away their business. In my opinion, there's enough business out there to go around for everybody. It's interesting that they feel threatened. Is it because the midwives can do a better job? Is it because they do it for less money? I don't know.'

The second key to success, she said, is the programme of home visits by public-health nurses. 'When our clients get back in their home setting, there are always issues that can't be addressed in a clinic or hospital, or in routine postpartum care. The home-visit nurses discuss things with the new mothers like how they're mixing their formula, the way they are taking care of their babies. The mothers suffer from information overload in the hospital and in the clinic; there are some things that need to be addressed personally in the home situation that can't be covered in the hospital.'

* My meeting with Martha Jinright was in March 1990. State health department statistics show that for the year 1990 there were 3,861 births in Montgomery County, of which Gift of Life delivered more than 1,600. In the first six months of 1991, Gift of Life delivered 738 babies. It would seem that Gift of Life is responsible for almost half of the births in Montgomery County.

The third ingredient in the Gift of Life's unique mix of services is what Doris Barnette described to me as 'case management', via the social services. 'This gives our clients a support mechanism, and someone they can call on for all kinds of help,' Ms Jinright said. 'Not somebody who just measures their bellies and addresses their clinical needs in prenatal care, but someone who can assist them when they may have some emotional problems. Everything from stress, to coping, to "I have a husband who's beating me on the weekends."

'Then we have some ladies who are so poor, homeless, with basic needs: "I have no food. I have nothing for my baby. It's thirty-two degrees outside and I have no blankets."' Inspired by the Gift of Life organisation, the community responded with 'food, bibs, bottles – what they call care packages. We've had a church use an old-fashioned pattern and make us some baby beds out of boxes. I know that some people think that's primaeval, but some of these ladies have no place for their babies. The boxes are darling. They cover them with pretty wallpaper, donate pillows and handsewn pillowcases.'

Doris Barnette had told me that the Gift of Life Foundation's board of directors range from ultra-liberal – a black former aide to Martin Luther King, Jr – to a white deep-dyed-conservative state senator. Martha Jinright elaborated: 'We have fourteen board members, six of whom are black. Part of the fascination, I think, about the foundation and its origination is that these people were able to come together for a common goal. I think that in itself is a major accomplishment, particularly in the South.' The black members include a member of the Board of Education, the dean of the black business college, and other community leaders. Do these work harmoniously with the white conservatives? I asked. 'Yes. Although they may be adversaries on other issues, they work very harmoniously on our board.'*

---

* Listening to Doris Barnette, Martha Jinright, John Porter, and numerous co-workers, I might have been lulled into forgetting that I was in the Cradle of the Confederacy had it not been for a chance encounter with one of the paediatric nurses, who delivered a prototypically racist spiel about the patients she is supposed to serve. She assured me that her views are shared by all her friends, and by extension by a majority of whites in Alabama. I suspect she may be right about this. In essence,

From these discussions, I gathered that the only way to reach into the hard hearts and shrivelled souls of the Alabama old-line politicians is via the path suggested in the *Journal* series, viz., to play upon their embarrassment when Alabama is tagged as 'the worst' place in the country to have a baby – even worse than Mississippi. Stalwarts in the Gift of Life programme, well aware of this, have learned to fine-tune their approach to the powerful to jangle that particular sensitive nerve.

Brave little Dutch boys with fingers in the dyke, the Gift of Life workers have counterparts elsewhere, individuals who are dedicated to the well-being of mothers and their babies and who use great ingenuity – carrots and sticks, cajolery and threats – to get around the sloth, inefficiency, and miserliness of government and its officials in bureaucracies from Medicaid to local boards of health.

Those most closely involved with the day-to-day work of these programmes have come to the inevitable conclusion that their efforts can only be a stopgap – a useful Band-Aid, but not a final solution to a huge and overriding problem.

Talking this over with Doris Barnette, I mentioned that the Netherlands, like most European countries, provides complete, free, comprehensive care for pregnant women, babies, and children, including everything from an adequate diet to midwifery and medical and paediatric services. If a Dutch child aged anywhere from three to ten is examined by health experts for such indicators as weight, height, and IQ, it is impossible to tell from these data whether the child comes from a rich, middle-class, or poor family, as he or she would have been entitled to all components of a healthy life regardless of financial status.

'That's a country that values its children regardless of their origin, because they are the future,' Mrs Barnette said, 'and I think one could draw the conclusion based on the system we have here, although it sounds like a real indictment, that perhaps we value only

she thinks that black teenagers should be penalised for having babies, should be denied prenatal care and cut off from welfare or any other assistance. 'Otherwise, two generations from now *my* grandchildren will be paying for the upkeep of *their* grandchildren, and on and on,' the nurse said, casting her pretty blue eyes skyward at the exasperating thought.

middle- and upper-income children. The data are there to tell us this is so.'

I asked Martha Jinright what she would think of a programme for the United States akin to those of the UK and Canada – a tax-supported national health service, providing free care to all. 'I'm not so sure I agree with socialised medicine across the board,' she said. 'But I think, because of the maternity-care crisis we have in this nation, we could learn a lot from socialised medicine in addressing the obstetrical situation.'

So it seems that from coast to coast those on the front line of maternity care – Drs Allen and Jackson in California, Doris Barnette and Martha Jinright two thousand miles away in Alabama – are of like minds when it comes to the root cause of the ever-escalating crisis. If their energies, and those of health workers across the country, could be mobilised for a concerted push towards national legislation that would ensure free access to decent health care for all citizens, we might yet see some revolutionary changes.

PART THREE

Doctors and Hospitals

Chapter 5

OBSTETRICIANS

In a letter to *The New York Times Book Review* of April 7, 1991, Diane J. Madlon-Kay, MD, drew attention to an interesting series of index entries in *Williams Obstetrics*, a classic textbook widely used by physicians and medical students. Apparently a feminist gremlin was at work during the boring task of preparing the index. Dr Madlon-Kay wrote: 'The index of the 15th edition, published in 1976, included a new heading: "Chauvinism, male, variable amounts, pages 1–923"'. The heading in the longer 16th edition of 1980 was altered conformably to read: 'Chauvinism, male, voluminous amounts, pages 1–1102.'

Did some 'chauvinist, male' editor spot it? In any event, the entry mysteriously disappeared from the 17th edition of 1985, Dr Madlon-Kay told us, adding caustically, 'Whether "Chauvinism, male" was also deleted from the text itself is debatable.'

Be that as it may, it would seem that 'Chauvinism, male' is endemic amongst medical students and fledgling physicians who have chosen to specialise in obstetrics. During the mid-1970s Diana Scully, a sociologist, spent three years as an observer in two hospitals with training programmes in obstetrics and gynaecology, watching procedures in the maternity wards and recording the conversations of residents, as these specialists-in-training are called. Among them, she soon discovered, there is also plenty of 'Chauvinism, racial' and 'Chauvinism, class'.

This was particularly noticeable in the Elite Medical Center (a pseudonym) in New England, where 60 per cent of the OB/GYN patients were private ones, mostly white, middle- and upper-class women; 40 per cent were 'institutional', black, working-class, poor. Care of the latter group was largely turned over to the residents, who were overwhelmingly white, male, from professional families, attracted to Elite because of its prestige.

After they got accustomed to Ms Scully's presence as a permanent fixture at Elite, the residents became almost disarmingly frank in discussing their career goals, what they hoped to accomplish during their four-year residencies, and their feelings about the OB/GYN patients.

Headed for a lucrative future in private practice, in which they would deal exclusively with paying patients, the residents saw their stint at Elite as simply a necessary learning experience; they believed their main job was to master as quickly as possible all the needed techniques to become full-fledged OB/GYN specialists. As one resident expressed himself in an interview with Scully:

> As far as I am concerned, my major responsibility is to get my education at this point, and my responsibility for providing patient care for the hospital or community is really quite negligible as far as I am concerned, but I have to give that in order to get my education.

Another told Scully:

> I know that in the first year I wanted to do as many forceps as possible, and this is just because of the selfish idea that I need the training. Everything is in case I need it. Part of being a doctor is the buildup of a very tough layer of skin, a very thick layer of confidence in yourself.

A resident looking ahead to better days said:

> You serve a different purpose in a private practice. You are a father image or a friend or something like that. Here we don't give that kind of service to the patients, they don't expect it. A lot of what you do in private practice is that, plus figure out what you are going to do with your money, trying to make money.

Opportunities to perform surgery were eagerly sought by the residents as essential to learning the skills of their profession and eventually entering private practice. They would haunt the clinic where the indigent patients went for prenatal care, or the evening family-planning sessions, and prowl around the emergency room looking for likely subjects. One resident proudly showed Ms Scully twelve pages of the names and telephone numbers of women who might be candidates for surgery. He would pursue these at leisure, even if there was no compelling medical reason for operating.

For example, if an examination showed that a woman had benign uterine fibroids, a condition that often does not require surgery, the art of persuasion would come into play – a cunningly designed sales pitch, reported in an interview at Elite:

> You have to look for your surgical procedures, you have to go after patients. Because no one is crazy enough to come and say, hey, here I am, I want you to operate on me. You have to some-times convince the patient that she is really sick, and that she is better off with a surgical procedure.

The private patients, likely to be sophisticated and well versed in trendy childbirth literature, had almost all taken Lamaze classes. They suffered pain, but tended to be more controlled and to scream less than their institutional sisters. The institutional patients couldn't afford the Lamaze classes; many of them didn't have husbands to participate in the delivery. 'Over and over, residents told me they disliked institutional patients; especially young, unmarried black women who lost control during delivery were a source of scorn,' Diana Scully reported. Some interviews bearing out this view:

> It is very difficult to deal with the institutional patients. I don't plan to have them in private practice. I don't plan to have a lot of 14- to 15-year-old girls that are pregnant in my office.

> It's a lot easier to take care of somebody that you can relate to – uh – I suppose that living a relatively sheltered existence, at least in terms of the people that I came into contact with, I really didn't have any close contact with the kind of people that come to Elite clinic . . .

I think basically I don't like to deal with uneducated people. They are people that know it is going to hurt and just start yelling from the beginning.

You know there are some people that you like and some people you can't stand ... If I like a patient, I will just automatically spend more time ... If somebody is over there screaming and raising hell, somebody that I don't like, they are just going to lay there ...

It's a personality thing, and with the institutional patients, you don't have anything to say about it, you have to take care of them. If you don't like the patient and they don't like you, they don't get taken care of properly.

Lest the foregoing should convey the idea that obstetricians are by nature and training uniformly avaricious, self-serving racists with no interest in the welfare of indigent patients, I should quickly say that this is by no means the whole picture. There is many a good apple in that barrel, drawn to the practice by fascination with the birth process, a strong desire to help women through pregnancy and birth, and an uncommon lack of interest in financial rewards.

Such a one is Greg Troll, a family practitioner in the Santa Cruz, California area. His early background, as he described it to me, would seem to make him Least Likely to Succeed in the profession he eventually embraced.

In 1969, Greg, then aged nineteen, was living in Detroit, where he worked during the day in an auto factory and at night as a wall washer in a teaching hospital. Assigned to clean the walls of the delivery suite, he thought the treatment of women in labour 'was really brutal. It just went against the grain of how I felt things ought to be done. I can't explain it except – I developed sort of a feeling about the process of birth from just listening.'

He got married and with his pregnant wife, Susan, attended Lamaze classes. They found an old German doctor who agreed to deliver the baby at home – a painful memory: the labour lasted thirty-three hours, the Lamaze 'monitrice'-cum-labour/delivery nurse, supposed to be a 'labour coach', was no help and spent most of the time sleeping.

Greg and Susan moved to Palo Alto, California, where in yet another career change he became a baker. In the early seventies their second child was born at home with a midwife attending. This time, the experience was so satisfactory that Susan decided to become a midwife. Greg studied along with her. 'I got really interested in it, I really wanted to do it. I didn't know any men who were into lay midwifery. It was, practically speaking, unheard of. Not only was it a total sex role novelty, but it was just strange.' Strange enough, it seems, so that the local midwives' collective refused to accept Greg as an apprentice because 'they didn't believe that men should be involved in birth'. Eventually he persuaded a midwife in the Santa Cruz area to take him on as a trainee. He decided to go to college as an undergraduate at the University of California, Santa Cruz, meanwhile attending many home births.

'At that point I sort of got in the direction of going to medical school, so I applied and was told I could forget it, I was too old and had too bizarre of a background.' One can almost sympathise with an admissions officer confronted with a résumé listing as occupations factory worker, wall washer, baker – a barber-surgeon, could one have been resurrected from medieval times, would have seemed more qualified. However, persistence paid off and Greg was admitted to Stanford University School of Medicine; he put in two years of classroom study, during which time as a lay midwife he continued to attend births of friends and fellow students, and a third year as a clerk in the Stanford hospital.

Having finished medical school, Greg – now Dr Troll – did his residency in Salinas at Natividad Medical Center, a county hospital as different from Diana Scully's 'Elite' as chalk from cheese. The patients in this farming community were almost all low-income, high-risk Mexican immigrants, many of whom spoke no English. 'We had drug addicts, diabetics; we had grand multigravidas, meaning women who have had thirteen, sixteen, seventeen pregnancies, other complications of pregnancy,' Greg said. 'The women who spoke Spanish came from rural areas in Mexico, and were, by and large, more comfortable with their bodies, more comfortable with labour and delivery. They didn't tend to be Lamazey, they weren't huffing and blowing. There's a lot of "*aie, aie, aie!*" – demonstrative complaining. They express their pain, and you stand by to be supportive, explain what's going on if necessary, and they deliver the baby. They did fine, by and large, those women.'

Greg's fellow residents were 'young, very idealistic people', he said, much given to group meetings where they discussed problems of individual patients, and reviewed in detail cases where it had been necessary to resort to medical intervention – specifically, Caesareans.

Some years before the American College of Obstetricians and Gynecologists issued its 1988 press release deploring the overuse of Caesareans, this was already a hot issue in obstetrics. A student survey of several hospitals in Greg's area revealed that the proportion of C-sections in private hospitals ran at about 30 per cent, the highest in 'an extremely swanky hospital on the Monterey Peninsula. It's the fanciest, looks like an art museum, with chamber music in the atrium. The Hilton of hospitals, with a C-section rate of 32 per cent.'

At the same time in Natividad Medical Center, with the highest-risk population of any of these hospitals, the rate ran between 17 and 19 per cent. This is a pattern often found in teaching hospitals, which, Greg said, tend to have a lower C-section rate. 'Possibly it's because people are more likely to question the procedure in each case, to ask each other, "Why are you going to do a section?" "Why did you do that section?" "What were your indications?"'

Nothing of the sort goes on in private hospital 'peer review' sessions, where the doctors function as an old boys' club. 'They get together once a month and review their cases. Somebody may say, "Yeah, she just wasn't progressing, so I sectioned her," and everyone will nod their head. No one is going to ask, "Well, let me see the foetal monitor strip," and "What was your indication there?" Not unless they have some political axe to grind against that person, and then they use everything they can against them; but in general, they're not going to. The general feeling is "If I question you on why you do a section, well, you might question me," and it makes life more complicated.'

Since Diana Scully's sojourn in obstetrical wards of the mid-1970s, there has been a dramatic change in the demographics of the profession, shown in statistics released by the American College of

Obstetricians and Gynecologists (ACOG). Over a fifteen-year period, 1976 to 1991, women have been making increasing inroads into the heretofore virtually all-male sanctum of OB/GYN. For example, in 1975–76, 16 per cent of first-year residents in the specialty were female; in 1990–91, 49 per cent. In 1975–76, 5.5 per cent completed a four-year residency and became ACOG fellows; in 1990–91, this rose to 20.5 per cent. ACOG adds that 'projections indicate that by the year 2000, 26 per cent of all OB/GYN practitioners will be women'.

The sudden influx of women into obstetrics was, by their own account, largely a by-product of the feminist movement of the 1960s and 1970s. What has been the day-to-day experience of women with the strength and tenacity to breach the masculine stronghold of the medical world? As described by my informants, it has been something like travelling through the bleak landscape of Bunyan's *Pilgrim's Progress*: the Slough of Despond, the Hill called Difficulty, the Valley of Humiliation.

Dr Rhoda Nussbaum, head of obstetrics at Kaiser Permanente in San Francisco, had been fascinated by medicine and biology since her childhood, when she watched shows about these subjects on television. 'But I was a little girl,' she said, 'and I think that in my family, with their background, I was supposed to *marry* a doctor, not *become* one.' So she settled for a career in physiotherapy, which she practised for two years until, in the late 1960s, she became immersed in the women's movement and, egged on by the sisterhood, decided to become a physician.

After returning to college to fulfill the undergraduate requirements, she applied to several medical schools. 'I was asked many times in interviews, "Are you married? When are you going to have a baby? What does your husband think of this?"' She was rejected by the American medical schools, and went to a medical school in Liège, Belgium, for two years. Back in America, having done exceptionally well on the standardised test required for entering students, she was accepted at the medical school of the University of Miami, after three years of which she entered the residency programme at Kaiser.

'I chose the GYN/OBS specialty because it is involved with women

– I am a feminist, so that was an attraction,' she said. And what about male practitioners in this field? I asked.

'My impression of gynaecologists, as a woman going to one in my teenage years and early twenties, and later my encounters with them in medical school, is that there were an awful lot of gynaecologists who were misogynists, who seemed to have chosen that field as a way to act out their dislike for women. I believe that's true. It's a sweeping generalisation, but that was my experience. But I should add that the year I was chief resident at Kaiser we had one male resident who doesn't fit that stereotype at all. I think he's responsible for lifting the quality of the department.'

Another who slogged her way through the Slough of Despond and up the Hill called Difficulty was Lisa Keller, a senior obstetrician/gynaecologist who now shares a private practice in Oakland with one other doctor, two certified nurse-midwives, and two nurse-practitioners.

In 1971, at the age of nineteen, she was a student at the University of California, Berkeley. Working as a volunteer at the Berkeley Free Clinic, she helped to organise a health collective patterned after the pioneering Boston Women's Health Book Collective, authors of *Our Bodies, Ourselves*. She had considered training as a nurse – like Rhoda Nussbaum, she was intimidated at the thought of becoming a doctor; but the support of her fellow activists convinced her to try.

'I applied to about ten medical schools and was accepted by three,' she told me. 'I finally decided on the University of California in Davis, where I went in 1979. There had been a big jump in women's enrolment there, from about seven per cent in 1971 to thirty per cent in my class.'

But even with this shift in the male/female ratio, the unspoken fact remained, reinforced by not-so-subtle reminders, that it was still a man's world. During Dr Keller's residency women were *ipso facto* shut out of the informal give and take of information by the simple device of a locker room for men only; the women doctors were restricted to the nurses' lounge.

'We were perfectly happy to be with the nurses,' she said. 'But on the other hand, if you wanted to get into what are the plans for tomorrow's conference, or how should I get paid for this job I'm going to do – those discussions are held in the men's place, and there's just no room for you there. You are just automatically excluded from all sorts of casual talk that happens in the men's locker room. I guess they call it the glass ceiling. A lot of it was that.'

Without a doubt, 1991 will go down in history as the year when sexual harassment in the workplace suddenly became Topic A in the popular press, as women who had suffered in silence from all manner of indignities began to declaim publicly against their treatment by male colleagues. Best remembered for initiating a nationwide debate on the issue may be Professor Anita Hill for her testimony against Judge Clarence Thomas (aka Long Dong Silver, with a pubic hair atop his can of Coke) in the Senate confirmation hearings of October.

Professor Hill was, however, preceded in June of that year by Dr Frances Conley, tenured professor of neurosurgery at Stanford University Medical School, where she had worked for twenty-three years, who resigned her post and loosed a stinging indictment of her male co-workers. 'Those who administer my work environment have never been able to accept me as an equal person,' she wrote. 'Not because I lack professional competence, but because I use a different bathroom. I am minus the appropriate gender identification that permits full club membership . . . even today, faculty are using slides of *Playboy* centerfolds to "spice up" lectures; sexist comments are frequent and those who are offended are told to be "less sensitive"; unsolicited touching and fondling occur between house staff and students. To complain might affect a performance evaluation.' And she told the press, 'I can't tell you how many times I have had some doctor run his hand up my leg.'

Which brings us to Bunyan's Valley of Humiliation. Apparently great minds think alike, in medical schools as elsewhere; to me, an intriguing phenomenon was the repetition from coast to coast – California to Connecticut – of a singularly idiotic joke played by male physicians to embarrass their female counterparts: displaying *Playboy* centrefolds, and flashing funny breast pictures on the screen during slide lectures. Sometimes the women lashed back. Some examples:

Dr Lisa Keller in California told me, 'There are still plenty of

pictures of women with bare breasts in the slides, thrown in out of
context in medical lectures, and stupid jokes about women – it's a
daily occurrence. And these were by physicians, grown-ups, who
supposedly knew better. In my supervisor's office there were always
Playboy pictures of bare-breasted women up on the wall. He said,
"Well, what's the matter with it?" He was grinning. "That's a pretty
woman up on the wall" – that sort of attitude. I asked him how
would he feel if there was a picture of a naked man with a big erection
on the wall. It was a sort of shock therapy; he'd go, "Oh well,
humph . . ."'

Dr Keller said that like Frances Conley she had undergone some
personal sexual harassment, but she managed to fend it off 'partly
because I am sort of aggressive and outgoing and I would just tell
them, "Oh, bug off" or be playful and flirt back. I think the more
shy women actually in some ways had it worse, because when men
see weakness they go for it.'

Dr Diane Barnes, a radiologist now in private practice, describing
her experience at Yale Medical School, told *The San Francisco Examiner*: 'We were constantly annoyed by a professor who punctuated
his lectures with a cartoon of "fifty different types of breasts and fifty
different slang names". So the women students in 1973, during the
annual freshman skit for parents, offered a slide show depicting male
genitals with fifty different slang names. And that was all we needed
to say. That slide on breasts never appeared again.'

In the *Western Journal of Medicine* of November 1991, Dr Linda
Hawes Clever, editor, set forth a bill of particulars that neatly summarised the indignities and hardships endured by her female co-
practitioners. It was a surprise to read this in an official publication
of the California Medical Association:

It has not been an easy road. Women physicians have endured
comments, jokes, prods, and worse. Some have been passed over,
ignored, dismissed. My internship in the 1960s was marred when
I was slapped in the face by a professor because I could not answer
his question. I did not report the incident. It didn't occur to me
to do so. Even today, as women contend with covert or overt
discrimination, most do not or cannot speak out.

. . . Leaders inside and outside medical schools have been slow or unwilling to set standards to make sexist barbs and practices wholly unacceptable . . .

How have women physicians weathered tough times and unfairness? We have had support from family, friends, and colleagues. We haven't complained much. Complaining wouldn't be seemly; it would also be a career-limiting activity.

. . . We have learned to be highly organized coordinators and jugglers, even jesters. A sense of humor can wear thin, however.

To what extent has the unprecedented entry of women into obstetrics influenced the profession as a whole, and specifically what impact have the female obstetricians had on the treatment of their patients?

Lisa Keller's response: 'Ah, that is the big question. In the past ten years women have become a factor in OB/GYN, but are still not breaking the male domination.

'I feel disappointment in women's overall lack of leadership, and failure to take the opportunity to change the medical mentality. I've been out of residency for ten years now. Women just two or three years ahead of me were just making it, in terms of personally making it in a terrible men's club. Women OB/GYN's haven't as yet made much of an impact on the profession; it is still almost entirely white, male-dominated, although conditions for the women doctors have improved since more are entering the practice.'

Dr Don Creevy, assistant professor of obstetrics at Stanford University School of Medicine, is a political progressive who has frequently tangled with other faculty members over such controversial issues as direct-entry midwives, for whom he is an ardent advocate, and home birth. Commenting on the new wave of women obstetricians in an interview with me on June 24, 1991, he recalled his own student days: 'When I was in medical school in Minneapolis, 1961 to '62, there were only four women in my class out of one hundred forty students, and when I was in residency at Stanford for four years there were no female residents. Now the Stanford residency programme in obstetrics runs roughly fifty-fifty, females and males.'

What about 'Chauvinism, male'? I asked.

'I think male chauvinism is rampant in medicine even today, and there have been numerous incidents at Stanford in the Department of Gynecology and Obstetrics.

'In order for a woman to get into medical school, to get through medical school successfully, to get into a specialty residency and complete that successfully, she's had to be a more than passingly aggressive woman. And I think that's led to a lot of female obstetricians being very aggressive and dominating ... So some of the female obstetricians I've known have been liberated women, but they certainly haven't encouraged their patients to be liberated. They continue in the sort of male-dominated spirit of things.

'Some of them I characterise as being more chauvinistic than the males are. But with this flood of women into the field I am seeing more and more women in obstetrics who are soft and gentle and kind and empathetic and supportive of women. The situation is improving.'

Chapter 6

ELECTRONIC FOETAL MONITORS AND ULTRASOUND

In *Dead Ringers*, a 1988 movie directed by David Cronenberg about identical twins who are brilliant and deranged gynaecologists (both acted by Jeremy Irons), there is a telling moment. We've been treated to a display of sinister-looking surgical implements invented by one of these brothers. We see one of them using a device resembling an instrument of torture on a terrified, agonised young woman. He exclaims in frustration, 'There's nothing the matter with the instrument – it's the body. The woman's body is all wrong.'

The same could be said of some of the innovative scientific paraphernalia and techniques that for the past many decades have been indispensable adjuncts to the practice of obstetrics; the instruments were fine, but somehow the bodies failed to respond correctly. The electronic foetal monitor is a case in point.

One of the most heartfelt objections to their hospital experience by mothers whose babies were born in the 1970s and 1980s was their coerced endurance of this new tool of the obstetrician's trade. The 'lithotomy position', in which the labouring woman is strapped supine in her narrow bed, pioneered by Joseph De Lee and denounced by correspondents to *The Ladies' Home Journal* as early as 1955, had long been the physicians' choice. In the 1970s there was added yet another cross to bear, in the shape of the electronic foetal monitor, a machine that electronically records the foetal heart rate during labour. In external foetal monitoring the abdomen is encircled by bands equipped with devices to record the baby's heart rate. The internal foetal monitor has two parts: an electrode that is screwed into the baby's scalp and records the heartbeat, and a catheter that lies alongside the baby and records the contractions of the uterus. The heartbeats and the contractions are shown separately on the monitor screen as graphs.

But supposing one screams out (as I think I would have, had anybody suggested such a procedure to me): 'You're not to put screws into my baby's head!' The definitively persuasive answer would be, 'But don't you want what's best for Baby? You want a healthy child, don't you? This is for *its* sake . . .'

Once the external monitor is in place, there can be no squirming around or shifting of position. The labouring woman must lie stockstill for fear of detaching the delicate machine, allegedly essential to her baby's well-being, which is recording every heartbeat on a printout like a stock-market ticker tape, in a remote nurses' station. Also, as the mother-to-be can't move to eat or drink, she is further encumbered by an IV (intravenous feeding tube) containing fluids, vitamins, etc., as well as, if ordered by the doctor, Pitocin to speed up the labour – this, ironically, because the enforced immobility of the woman may have caused labour to slow or indeed stop altogether.

While feminist authors whose books on childbirth I have consulted grumble plenty about foetal monitoring, questioning whether the information retrieved can be any more reliable than that available to the attentive midwife equipped with a stethoscope, medical researchers have only recently addressed the subject. Their findings, based on those ubiquitous 'studies' beloved by the scientific community, would seem to have put quietus to any future use of the monitors.

I first learned about this development from an unlikely source: a squib in *The Irish Times* of February 25, 1991, headlined 'Foetal Heart Monitoring Discarded', by Dr Robert Simpson. He cited an address by Sir Donald Acheson to the Royal College of Midwives in London which contended: 'Continuous monitoring of the baby's heart during labour may soon be a thing of the past,' and he quoted the American College of Obstetricians and Gynecologists as saying that electronic foetal heart monitors 'are not worthwhile'. Simpson concluded that 'the age-old tradition of the midwife listening to the baby's heart through the mother's abdominal wall with an ear trumpet will continue'.

The ear trumpet, mentioned nowhere in the medical lit, was, I thought, a charming idea, so I sent the clipping to Dr Warren Pearse, director of the American College of Obstetricians and Gynecologists, in Washington, DC, for further clarification. His reply, in a letter dated March 31, 1991: 'ACOG's judgment is not that EFMs are "not worthwhile", but that for low-risk situations they do not offer outcome advantages over auscultation via stethoscope.' (Auscultation, by the way, means listening; but why use a short word when a longer one is available?)

He enclosed ACOG Technical Bulletin 132, September 1989, which restated the original goal of the EFM – detection of danger signs 'in time to permit intervention' – and which went on to say, 'Previously, it had been presumed that continuous electronic foetal monitoring would be more sensitive and accurate than intermittent auscultation . . . This presumption has not been supported by recent studies.' Well I never. That was some 'presumption', causing a whole generation of childbearing women to submit to this marvellous, indisputably accurate, lifesaving product of the finest brains in the medical scientific community. The ACOG bulletin added: 'Retrospective reports suggested the benefit of continuous electronic foetal monitoring, and this type of monitoring was urged for all women in labour.' It concluded: 'A significant increase in the rate of operative deliveries, both vaginal and abdominal, was reported in women who received continuous electronic foetal monitoring . . . Caesarean delivery rate was also significantly increased.'

How and why did this phenomenon gain such a prominent place in the American maternity ward? The best and most authoritative account of its origins, rise, and probable fall was set forth in an article titled 'Whither Electronic Monitoring?' by Herbert F. Sandmire, in *Obstetrics and Gynecology*, December 1990.

Straight off, we learn that the initial introduction of the EFM was 'largely based on promising animal studies'. But as Lotte Lenya sang in Kurt Weill's *Mahagonny*, 'ein Mensch ist kein Tier', or in plain English, 'A man is not an animal'; nor is a woman, it turns out.

First developed in the 1960s, by the early 1970s continuous electronic foetal monitoring not only became the standard of care for high-risk patients, but 'this unproved technology was widely applied to low-risk patients as well. Unfortunately, after almost 20 years of experience, it is now apparent that the anticipated benefits to the foetus, newborn and child have not materialised.'

Disadvantages of electronic foetal monitoring, Sandmire wrote, include an increase in Caesarean deliveries, leading to a substantial increase in maternal illness and death; higher costs for obstetrical care; and legal risks for the attending physician, with nearly half of all obstetrical liability claims involving EFM. Sandmire suggested that labouring patients should, at a minimum, receive information to allow them to make an informed choice between EFM and the stethoscope for keeping track of the unborn infant's heartbeat.

And this from down under: Australian physicians Paul B. Coditz and David J. Henderson-Smart of King George V Hospital for Mothers and Babies, Camperdown, New South Wales, wrote in 1990: 'Intrapartum electronic monitoring of the foetal heart rate and acid-base status* have not been shown to prevent asphyxia or cerebral palsy . . . Data from several studies of large numbers of pregnancies suggest that high risk foetuses who receive intrapartum continuous electronic heart rate monitoring do not have a better outcome than those who receive monitoring by intermittent auscultation of the heart rate.' The authors concluded that intermittent checking of the foetal heart rate via stethoscope is just as safe a method, and added, 'This will at least ensure that the primary focus of the obstetric personnel will be the mother and her baby rather than an electronic monitor.'

Incidentally, the belated acknowledgment by the medical scientific community of the shortcomings – and deleterious effects – of the electronic foetal monitors merely repeats what midwives have been saying all along. When they denounced the monitors as harmful,

---

* As the oxygen in the baby's blood decreases, the acidity increases. The measurement of acidity is used to assess the stress caused by lack of oxygen.

pointing out that one intervention inexorably leads to others, citing the increase in C-sections, they were roundly condemned by the medical establishment as ignorant know-nothings.

Akin to the electronic foetal monitor is ultrasonography, the use of diagnostic ultrasound at intervals throughout pregnancy, supposedly to reveal not only the length of gestation and estimated date of birth, but also such complications as the existence of twins. Formerly these matters were determined by X rays, long discontinued – and just as well. A friend of mine, pregnant circa 1944, got unusually huge toward the end of her term. Twins seemed to be the likely reason, so her doctor ordered X rays. When the pictures came back, he told her that the photos showed 'multiple limbs, but only one head'. For the next two weeks she suffered through the dismal thought of giving birth to a humanoid starfish, but in the event perfectly healthy well-formed twins emerged.

Everyone now knows that X rays are harmful, never to be used on pregnant women. How about ultrasound? Is it safe, is it useful for its purpose? As to safety, nobody really knows; it is too soon to tell. Nervous early warnings have been issued by medical sceptics. Thus Sheila Kitzinger wrote in 1980 that 'no one yet knows if any of them (babies) will suffer delayed effects in later life'. Robert Mendelsohn, in his illuminating book *How to Raise a Healthy Child in Spite of Your Doctor* (New York: Ballantine, 1987) said that the use of ultrasound for diagnosis 'raises some alarming questions that can't be answered by those who employ it'. There is no conclusive evidence linking ultrasound to foetal damage, he said, 'nor is there any hard evidence that it will not cause damage. In short, I can't prove conclusively that ultrasound may damage your baby, but the doctor who uses it on you can't prove that it won't.'

As for its diagnostic usefulness, in August 1990, *Obstetrics and Gynecology* published an exhaustive study of pregnant women examined by this method for estimated date of confinement and for possible twins. The conclusion: 'There was no benefit found from routine ultrasound as performed in this study.'

In 1985 the Royal Society of Medicine in London conducted a

forum on ultrasonography in obstetrics, and published its findings the following year. None of the six speakers at this prestigious gathering had a kind word to say for the routine use of ultrasound – on the contrary, they betrayed considerable uneasiness about its as yet unproven safety.

The lead-off speaker, Dr Ann Oakley of the University of London's Institute of Education, noted that by the late 1970s, ultrasound foetal surveillance had become commonplace in many countries – especially those with insurance-based health care systems: 'Indeed, commercial interests are essential to consider when trying to understand the spread of a new technique, although it is extremely difficult to acquire reliable information on these interests ... It is the rule rather than the exception that clinical practice absorbs new techniques on the basis of inadequate evidence of their effectiveness and safety.' She added: 'Advocates of a new technique are liable to suffer from a strange condition called certainty.'

Illustrating the strange condition, she cited passages from a standard textbook, *Antenatal and Postnatal Care*, on the subject of X rays. The 1937 edition stated with certainty, 'It has been frequently asked whether there is any danger to the life of the child by the passage of X rays through it; it can be said at once that there is none.' The same textbook in its 1960 edition, after the link between *in utero* X rays and childhood cancer had been well established, advised, 'It is now known that the unrestricted use of X rays may be harmful to mother and child.'

In Dr Oakley's view, the development of obstetrical ultrasound mirrors the application to human pregnancy of diagnostic X rays: 'In 1935 it was said that "antenatal work without the routine use of X rays is no more justifiable than would be the treatment of fractures." In 1978: "It can be stated without qualification that modern obstetrics and gynaecology cannot be practiced without the use of diagnostic ultrasound."'

For the obstetrician, ultrasonography can be an enjoyable pastime for what it tells about the life-style of a foetus: its breathing movements, hiccups, eye movements, how often it empties its bladder. 'This is doubtlessly fascinating work, but what is its ethical justification?' Dr Oakley asked. 'Are the women and foetuses involved in these studies (none of whom are getting it because they need it) informed that the long-term effects of ultrasound are unknown? Is what is learned from all this research likely to be of overall benefit to the welfare of the childbearing population?' Picking at random from studies focusing on foetal movements in pregnancy, Dr Oakley came across one which relayed in ponderous prose the discovery that 'the foetus does not always move in one and the same manner', that its behaviour is 'a complex of spontaneous movements and a motionless period between them'. She pointed out, 'Any mother can tell you that foetuses don't always move in the same way, and that sometimes a healthy foetus doesn't move at all; it sleeps like the rest of us.'

Dr Oakley poured scorn on the claim that ultrasound enables obstetricians to 'introduce' mothers to their foetuses, and 'facilitates a new phenomenon called prenatal bonding in exactly the same way that the medical innovation of hospital delivery enabled paediatricians to discover the phenomenon of postnatal bonding. I would suggest that this is just rediscovering-the-wheel of a most primitive kind. Mothers and newborns bonded before in-hospital delivery disturbed the natural process . . . They are in a relationship with each other before they meet on the ultrasound screen.'

In the discussion after Dr Oakley's presentation, a voice from the audience suggested that the routine use of ultrasound 'was being promoted by those who had purely financial motives'. Another audience member made the point that 'if all pregnancies were monitored with ultrasound, junior doctors would never acquire clinical monitoring skills, and those who already possessed them would lose confidence in their ability to learn by using their eyes, ears, and hands.'

Nancy Stewart, a representative of the Association for Improvement in the Maternity Services (based in Shropshire), told the gathering that the scan can be a frightening experience for the pregnant woman; some had reported that they weren't told anything about the scan's findings. It is an assembly-line procedure through which women are rushed by busy operators who haven't got time to explain anything. One woman was told, 'We can't find the baby's head. You'll have to come back next week.'

While debates about the safety of ultrasound have progressed in the professional journals, Ms Stewart said, 'women have consistently been assured that it is completely harmless. One doctor conceded that ultrasound cannot precisely be termed "harmless", yet wrote, "In the context of a doctor–patient relationship, this statement is not misleading." Many women resent being told that ultrasound is safe when the truth is that nobody knows.'

Chapter 7

FORCEPS

The use of forceps to prise the baby out of its hiding place has had a chequered history. In the eighteenth century William Hunter, a leading English accoucheur, declared that 'It was a thousand pities forceps were invented. Where they save one, they murder twenty.' The same thought, phrased in more circumspect language, was to re-emerge in the medical literature of the 1980s after routine forceps delivery for most births had once again fallen into disrepute.

By the mid-twentieth century forceps manufacture was in high gear, with many different models vying for the obstetrical trade. Looking over some of the offerings, vividly illustrated with line drawings, in *Williams Obstetrics* (seventeenth edition, 1985) I noticed that one can choose between 'Simpson Forceps . . . ample pelvic curve'; 'Tucker-McLane . . . solid blade, narrow shank'; 'Kielland forceps featuring sliding lock, lightweight'; 'Tarnier forceps, axis handle traction'; 'Barton forceps . . . sliding lock and one hinged blade', etc. It occurred to me that if the labouring woman were shown these pictures and the descriptions, and asked to state her preference, she might vote for none of the above. An unlikely scenario, because while delivery by forceps is described in the medical lit as an 'elective' procedure, there is no evidence that the mother-to-be was ever considered part of the voting constituency.

According to obstetricians I have consulted who practised in the 1950s, forceps delivery was the preferred method in at least 50 per cent of births. Dr James Jackson, now head of obstetrics at Highland Hospital in East Oakland, California, told me, 'I was trained to do episiotomies and forceps when I first went into practice and that's what I did. I thought that anaesthesia and episiotomy and forceps delivery were appropriate.' But routine use of forceps 'just sort of went by the board', he said. Today, out of 250 births a month, his department averages about two forceps deliveries.

Reliable statistics on the use of forceps nationwide in the peak years of the early 1950s are hard to come by – possibly they were unrecorded or unreported or both. Warren Pearse of ACOG told me in a letter dated May 13, 1991, that 'in the 1950s, rates of forceps delivery as reported by various hospitals ranged from two per cent to 50 per cent' – which is quite a range. He added that much depended on the type of anaesthesia: 'Epidural or spinal anaesthetic removes the expulsive powers in the second stage of labour and often necessitated forceps delivery.'

In an effort to clarify once and for all some of the highly confusing terms that occur throughout the medical texts, in May 1991 I consulted Dr Don Creevy, assistant professor of obstetrics at Stanford University School of Medicine, for some simple explanations, comprehensible to the layman – and even more to the point, to the laywoman.

What, precisely, is meant by the first, second, and third stages of labour? 'The first stage of labour begins when contractions are occurring regularly every five minutes or so, and there is progressive opening and thinning of the cervix, which is at the lower end of the uterus. It ends when the cervix is fully dilated, meaning approximately ten centimetres, and when one can no longer feel the cervix as a separate entity on vaginal examination. You feel the baby's head, but you feel no rim of tissue around the head.' And the second stage? 'I'll put it this way: from complete cervical dilation (ten centimetres) until delivery of the baby. Third stage is from delivery of the baby to delivery of the placenta.'

And what about forceps – high, mid, low? 'These refer to where the head is in the pelvis when the forceps are applied, not to a specific type of obstetrical forceps. High forceps means application of forceps when the baby's head has not yet dropped into the mother's pelvis. Low forceps: the baby's head is on the mother's pelvic floor, facing straight back toward the mother's spine. Mid forceps: the baby's head is engaged (has dropped into the pelvis) but is not on the pelvic floor and is not facing straight back.

'I was taught in medical school in the late 1950s that to apply high forceps was an obstetrical crime.' (The same idea is conveyed in *Williams Obstetrics:* 'High-forceps delivery has no place in modern obstetrics . . . and is mentioned here only to be condemned.')

High forceps, then, is no longer an issue in the obstetrical profession. The controversy that simmered from the 1950s to the 1980s had to do with mid and low forceps – when, or whether, to use these devices.

Don Creevy, who is not a fan of forceps, uses them very sparingly – 'The last time I looked at my statistics I did forceps deliveries about three per cent of the time. And my Caesarean rate is about six to seven per cent.' Forceps rotation, he explained, is the technique of using obstetrical forceps to turn the baby's head 'if it is facing in a direction that is not consistent with the ability to fit through the birth canal', for example if the head is facing toward the mother's abdomen rather than toward her spine, 'when they come out and fit best that way'. Manual rotation, just using the fingers to turn the baby into a normal position, may be a better and safer procedure: 'The problem with forceps rotation is that inadvertently you can damage the baby's head, and you can damage the mother's tissues.'

The latest available national data on forceps, Dr Pearse wrote to me, are from a 1980 survey which reported 15 per cent of deliveries by forceps and an 11 per cent C-section rate. 'Forceps deliveries have continued to decline for a number of reasons. In probable order of importance, these reasons are the increased rate of C-section, concerns about professional liability, fewer epidural anaesthetics, and the use of the vacuum extractor.' (The latter, perfected in 1954, consists of a metal or plastic cup that produces suction. *Williams Obstetrics* (seventeenth edition) says that 'in spite of early enthusiasm' it is not used widely because of foetal damage and deaths of infants, which seems like a sound enough reason.)

Medical opinion on forceps delivery, as reflected in the professional journals, has swung back and forth. In 'Midforceps Delivery – a Vanishing Art?' published in 1963, the authors contended that 'the dictum that midforceps delivery is obsolete and that it should be replaced by Caesarean section is a convenient platitude ... Too often today a potentially difficult labour is avoided by the over-enthusiastic use of C-section.'

The authors predicted dire consequences for their profession should the anti-forceps faction prevail:

> With such an approach to the problem one can foresee the horrible possibility of obstetricians consisting of midwives performing normal deliveries, and surgeons performing C-sections!
>
> ... The authors' title question, 'Midforceps, a vanishing art?' must be answered in the negative, so that it will not vanish and we may remain obstetricians, not midwives!

As we have seen, Dr De Lee, he of the spawning salmon analogy, was an ardent early advocate of forceps for *all* births, along with the lithotomy position, sedation from the first stage of labour, and episiotomy. Although De Lee died in 1942, his legacy lived on; in the Chicago Lying-In Hospital (where he had originally been in charge) in the years between 1946 and 1951 the rate of forceps delivery was 68.2 per cent. (How the other 31.8 per cent managed to elude the forceps must remain a matter of conjecture.)

One of Dr De Lee's many disciples, L. V. Dill, set forth the pro-forceps position in his book *The Obstetrical Forceps*, published in 1953 when use of the device was at its zenith. He noted:

> In many areas of the country at this time ... the use of forceps is routine for all or a large portion of vertex presentations [meaning the baby emerges head first] ... Its growth has been enhanced by extensive usage of analgesia and anesthesia which cause pro-longation of the second stage by inhibiting voluntary cooperation of the patient.

While the whole point of forceps was to speed up the second stage of labour, opinions differed as to just when they should be used. Dr Dill wrote, 'There are many individual variations. There are rules in some institutions that after a half-hour or a one-hour second stage, the forceps should be applied.' He said that while such a rigid clock-defined criterion is absurd, it's up to the individual doctor to decide in any given case when is the right moment for forceps. 'Gone are 'the days when forceps were used to deliver women who could be delivered vaginally only with the greatest difficulty, if at all,' he wrote, and he added in a burst of enthusiasm: 'It has truly become an instrument of "deliverance".'

There were voices of dissent. One who swam vigorously against the prevailing tide of medical opinion was E. Stewart Taylor in a 1953 article, 'Can Mid-Forceps Operations Be Eliminated?' His findings, based on thirty-one mid-forceps deliveries in two Colorado hospitals: 'Eight of the 31 mid-forceps operations resulted in still-born or injured infants that died from birth injury shortly thereafter. This represents a fetal mortality of 26 percent. There were an additional 7 infants who suffered birth trauma and lived,' for a total death and injury rate of 48 per cent for mid-forceps procedures. Aside from this large number of dead and damaged babies, the mothers didn't fare too well, as the mid-forceps 'produce undesirable damage to the maternal pelvic structure' and resulted in 'hemorrhage and shock in a high percentage of patients.'

(A comment here by Don Creevy: 'This is certainly *not* representative of carefully carried out mid-forceps deliveries. The MDs in his series must have been "poor users" or had poor judgment.')

Dr Taylor continued: 'If C-section had been elected . . . it is likely that 8 fetal deaths and the injuries to 7 infants would have been avoided.' He concluded that forceps operations 'carry a prohibitive fetal mortality and morbidity', and that they are 'rarely indicated in modern obstetrical practice'.

There were some nasty moments. In an interview published in his book *MD: Doctors Talk About Themselves* (New York: Dell, 1988) John Pekkanen recorded the following: 'The nurses reported an obstetrician who had put his foot against the delivery table and used that as leverage to extract a baby with forceps. You can rip a baby's head off if you pull too hard! The baby was damaged as a result of the unnecessary force he exerted in this delivery.'

The above horror story might be taken for an isolated incident concerning an unusually inept obstetrician, were it not for references to the same procedure in the medical literature. For example, Lamar Ekbladh wrote:

I was once told that a hard forceps delivery involves putting your feet up against the delivery table and pulling with all your might. Easy forceps means applying force with the forearms only. But how many of us can be certain when we're using other muscles besides our forearms? We may be guilty of labeling a delivery difficult or easy according to the outcome, not according to what we did.

A couple of comments on the above. From Don Creevy: 'To a man with a set of forceps in his hand, every baby's head looks as if it needs help being born!' And to a woman? From Rhoda Nussbaum, head of obstetrics at Kaiser Permanente in San Francisco: 'The majority of the residents in my programme are women whose body weight probably averages less than one hundred thirty pounds. Hard forceps – if defined by massive physical effort on the part of the OB – is ludicrous. I'm not strong enough to apply the kind of physical force described above.' She made a further point: 'Given that routine use of forceps or vacuum is bad – does that imply that all use is wrong? I think not. There are few but definite cases where use of this tool is extremely helpful.'

I asked Greg Troll, whose medical career spanned the decline and fall of the routine use of forceps, what his experience had been.

'One of the problems with tools of the trade is that when you have a tool you tend to use it,' he said. 'I did two hundred fifty births in a row and I never used forceps once, in an environment where everybody else thought that they had to use forceps twenty to thirty per cent of the time, in exactly the same patient population. And I had a lower Caesarean rate and a lower complication rate than they did.'

By the 1980s, the anti-forceps dissidents were gaining the upper hand in the professional journals – although to what extent these are read, absorbed, and acted on by practitioners is unknowable. (Greg Troll told me that obstetricians 'probably don't read these articles. My impression is that obstetricians are less scientific-minded than other medical specialists'.)

In their article 'Current Role of the Midforceps Operation', published in 1980, Watson A. Bowles and Christine Bowes, citing Taylor's finding of 1953, pointed out that more than twenty years ago it was known that mid-forceps operations carry definite hazards for mother and infant. Training resident physicians in the proper usage of mid forceps is difficult, they said: 'Teaching the technique to a neophyte is like instructing a new pilot to fly a plane with but one set of controls', as only one person at a time can apply the forceps, manoeuvre the blades, and exert the traction. A single resident may perform the operation only three or four times a year. Conversely, Caesareans can be easily taught; a junior resident may perform thirty to forty each year.

In a symposium documented in May 1980 four experts discussed the forceps issue. Emanuel Friedman, professor of OB/GYN at Harvard Medical School, led off by saying, 'I'm convinced that mid-forceps is an anachronism ... Long-term follow-up reveals a clear-cut relationship between mid-forceps use and speech, language, and hearing losses at age three, and lowered IQ scores at age four.' Babies delivered by forceps may have appeared normal, he said, but abnormalities began to show up by the time they were three to four years old. There was also a 'clear relationship between perinatal mortality and the use of instruments, particularly mid-forceps'.

Dr Michael J. Hughey of Northwestern University School of Medicine, citing an analysis of 470 patients going back to 1967, agreed: 'There was no question that the babies who had mid-forceps rotation did not do as well as those not subjected to the procedure.'

As to the major rationale for forceps delivery – the dangers supposedly inherent for mother and baby in unduly prolonged labour – the doctors unanimously declared that there was no factual basis to support this theory.

Thus Dr Lamar Ekbladh of Chapel Hill, North Carolina, asserted: 'It's passé to insist that the second stage must end after one or two hours.'

And Dr Friedman said:

A recent study at our institution showed that the duration of the second stage – even when greatly prolonged – had literally nothing to do with the outcome ... The increased perinatal mortality [meaning death of the infant shortly before or after birth] was the result of the intervention, not of prolonged second stage. The intervention can be far more damaging than time elapsed.

And what about vacuum extraction? 'It's not a viable alternative,' said Dr Friedman. 'It's subject to the same objections as are traction forceps.'

By the time of the symposium, in 1980, there was another factor to be reckoned with: a newfound determination by the maternity patients to be informed about procedures, and to have a say in what was to be done. As described by Dr Ekbladh:

> The trend is for the patient to be more involved in the labour and delivery process. She may no longer accept that she needs to be delivered after 1 or 2 hours in the second stage. She may ask, 'Is the baby having problems? If not, why do you have to do anything?' The patient expects that we will intervene only if she or her infant is at risk – and that we will keep her informed of whatever risks are inherent in what we do.

By about 1980, forceps were in steep decline – still used to some extent by experienced old-timers in especially difficult labours, but no longer considered appropriate for all comers. ACOG's nationwide survey of 1980, reporting 15 per cent forceps, 11 per cent Caesareans, foretold the shape of things to come: good-bye forceps, hello Caesareans.

Chapter 8

CAESAREANS

In a spectacular leap forward for the high-tech trendsetters in the obstetrical profession, by 1987 approximately one out of every four babies born in the United States was from its mother's womb untimely ripp'd, up from one in twenty in 1970. Everything was going along swimmingly for the C-section enthusiasts – C-sections rising at the rate of one per cent a year – until October 1988, when the American College of Obstetricians and Gynecologists issued its landmark bulletin advocating abandonment of the medical tenet 'Once a Caesarean, always a Caesarean' and urging the option of vaginal delivery for most women who had had a previous C-section. These accounted for one-third of all Caesarean births, hence were a significant factor in the unprecedented increase in the procedure. The ACOG statement was featured in newspapers nationwide. Soon, the initials VBAC, pronounced 'veebac' – meaning Vaginal Birth After Caesarean – reverberated throughout the land, heeded by some obstetricians, ignored by many. In any event, the rate had decreased slightly in 1989, for the first time in 25 years, from 24.7 per cent to 24.4 per cent, mostly attributable to VBACs, according to figures from the National Center for Health Statistics. Curiously, this information was only released two years later – in July 1991. National statistics on Caesareans, as on other medical matters such as the continued use of electronic foetal monitors – any change since ACOG's 1989 pronouncement of their relative worthlessness – are frustratingly either unavailable or some years behind. This seems odd, in the land of computerised information on every subject from the consumption of Twinkies to the rise and fall of real estate values.

*

The Caesarean operation has changed tremendously since it was first successfully performed by Max Sänger in the 1880s. In the early days, it must have been a pretty devastating experience for the mother: she spent hours under total anaesthetic while the doctor cut and sutured layers of skin and muscle; she remained bedridden and in pain for many weeks thereafter; and she was left with a huge permanent vertical scar that ran the length of her abdomen. But it was worth it, obviously, if she and the baby survived when one or both would otherwise have perished. For any subsequent births, she would certainly have been subjected to the same surgery, as there was danger of the scar in the uterine wall ripping apart if she should go through the strain of normal labour.

During the last many decades, the technique has improved beyond recognition. From the doctor's point of view, it is a simple operation that normally takes from twenty to forty-five minutes once everything is in place: patient, anaesthetist, and nurses all set to go. Instead of the debilitating general anaesthetic, a regional – spinal or epidural – may be given, in which case the baby's father is often allowed to stay and watch the Miracle of Birth, twentieth-century-style. Above all, the uterine incision is no longer the vertical cut of yore, known as 'classical' in the literature, but the 'low transverse'. This makes possible a crescent-shaped incision slightly below the pubic hairline – a considerable cosmetic improvement, sometimes called the 'bikini cut'. The healed scar is almost invisible and easily concealed by the briefest of those garments. Aside from that undeniable benefit, the operation itself is far safer; there is very small risk that the uterine scar would burst open in a subsequent vaginal birth.

In his 1989 book *The Cesarean Myth*, Dr Mortimer Rosen, head of OB/GYN at Presbyterian Medical Center and the College of Physicians and Surgeons, Columbia University, told us that 'the patient will inevitably face certain complications:

She won't be able to eat for a day or more.

She will be in considerable pain and will continue to have some pain for about six weeks; she will often find it painful to urinate, defecate, or move freely.

She will have a urinary bladder catheter for a day or so.

She will probably need painkillers.

She will have up to four or seven days' hospital stay.

She will have a good chance of developing some sort of infection, which will need antibiotic treatment.

And of course if she is a convinced believer in the unique experience of unmedicated, natural labour and birth, she will have missed all that; worse yet, she may get little enjoyment out of looking after her newborn, as she may be feeling too wretched to appreciate that pleasure.

While most mothers who deliver vaginally regain their normal energy by six weeks after the birth – 72 per cent, according to the Public Citizen Health Research Group (a spin-off from Ralph Nader's organisation) – only 34 per cent of Caesarean mothers feel they are back to normal after six weeks.

Wanting to find out how the whole procedure went for mothers who have been through it, I consulted several women who have had Caesareans in the last few years. While most of my respondents generally confirmed Mortimer Rosen's description of the post-operative miseries, there were variations – largely due, it seems, to the attitude of the attending obstetrician and hospital staff.

April Kubachka of Harbor City, California, was nineteen years old in 1984, when she had her first baby in a hospital. (She later learned that the hospital's Caesarean rate that year was 31.7 per cent, considerably above the national average.) I asked whether the doctor had explained to her the reason for a Caesarean, and if so whether she was satisfied with his explanation.

'I don't remember *any* doctor discussing it with me,' she answered. 'All I remember is a nurse telling me they were going to have to do an emergency C-section for foetal distress and she needed me to sign the consent form. No, it was *not* satisfactory.'

The operation lasted about an hour. 'I will never forget the intense pain I felt when the spinal anaesthetic had worn off,' Kubachka said. 'It was this continuous dull ache that never went away no matter what position I lay in. And I will never forget the pain of the "first walk", the morning after surgery. It took me at least three months to regain my normal energy level. I felt totally cheated – totally ripped off of my first birth experience; I felt the whole process of birth had been orchestrated by the medical staff instead of by my body.'

After twelve hours of labour she was three centimetres dilated, 'but that wasn't good enough for the hospital staff. Instead of confining me to bed strapped to a foetal monitor, they should have had me up and walking around. Instead of pumping me full of drugs they should have had me showering, eating lightly, and drinking fluids. It's no wonder that my son went into distress. I feel as though I was treated as a uterus with a baby inside.'

Ms Kubachka went home after three and a half days in the hospital, which included the twelve hours of labour before the operation. She asked to leave early because she had no medical insurance. The bill was another shock: for the hospital alone, $3,000. With doctor's and anaesthetist's fees, the total was over $5,000. (This of course was in 1984!)

Eventually she confronted her obstetrician, demanding to know the precise reason for the Caesarean. 'Because your son was in distress. We don't know what caused it.' He added significantly: 'We get hung for the Caesareans we *don't* do.'

Four years later Ms Kubachka, not much older but a lot wiser, decided on a VBAC for her next baby, scheduled for delivery at Kaiser Hospital in Bellflower. For this one, she planned to stay at home after labour started until the last minute, and she did: walking, taking a shower, eating toast and fruit juice, even spending some hours in a neighbour's Jacuzzi. Her husband, her sister, and a birth attendant hovered around helping, but the last minute came and went – the hospital was a thirty-minute drive from her house – and the baby, nicknamed for obvious reasons Freeway, was born in the backseat of the car en route. Ms Kubachka remembers it as an exhilarating and almost pain-free experience.

Sarah Pattee of San Diego was thirty-one when she had a Caesarean for the birth of her first child in 1988. She had planned a home birth, but was transported to a hospital (with C-section rate 33 per cent) when labour began to seem too long and arduous.

She told me, 'I experienced animosity from the nursing staff because I was a "failed home birth". One nurse went so far as to tell me that "pizza is for home delivery, not birth!" The cost was seventy-five hundred dollars, which still astounds me as I only stayed one day and two nights and kept my son with me the entire time. They still charged me two hundred fifty dollars for his one-night nursery stay, although he slept in my arms.

'You asked if the doctor discussed the reason for the Caesarean with me. I don't believe there is such a thing. Most women – and this includes me – are told, "The baby is in danger and we've got to get him out now!"'

After the epidural anaesthesia wore off, she said, 'I remember this excruciating fiery pain. I was left in a recovery room, looking like a dead fish left on the shore and feeling worse.'

She had trouble breast-feeding the baby because her scar was so raw and tender that she couldn't get into a comfortable position. In the hospital she developed a vaginal infection, and sustained damage to her urethra during catheterisation. For months after the surgery she suffered a deep depression: 'I cried, I raged,' she said. 'I still remember the pain of coughing, sneezing, laughing – I prayed I wouldn't do any of them.'

Like April Kubachka, Pattee was determined to avoid a repeat of this awful experience and decided on a VBAC – in her case, at home attended by a midwife, her husband, and a friend. She gave birth squatting on a rug. The baby slid out: 'I put her to my breast, she suckled and slept. What is amazing is that from three to five a.m. I was higher than a kite, calling my family in Europe ... I had so much energy and euphoria – what an incredible difference from my first birth!'

For Stacey Josted of Sacramento, whose two children, born in 1985 and 1989, were both delivered by unplanned Caesareans, the experience was entirely different from those described above. In each case, her obstetrician explained in detail his reason for rec-ommending the operation. 'Here is the real key,' she said. 'A decision-making process that involves the parents with the physician, and allows the parents to make the ultimate decision after receiving a complete and understandable review of *all* the options available to them.' The other important factor: '*Respect* for the birthing woman by the hospital staff. Wouldn't this make all hospital births better?'

Ms Josted believes that she was most fortunate in her choice of obstetricians, both of whom resist the mainstream 'medical model' of birth and are strong opponents of Caesareans unless there are – as in her case – compelling reasons. Her first was delivered by Don Creevy at Stanford University Hospital; her second, by Leon Schimmel at Woodland Memorial Hospital. Did she suffer much pain? 'Yes, particularly with the first one. I had significant pain for about a week, gradually lessening, but continuing for several months. There was pain at the incision site for over a year.'

All three of these women are today active workers in the Cesarean Prevention Movement, founded in 1982 by Esther Zorn of Syracuse, New York, herself the victim of an unnecessary, debilitating Caesarean for the birth of her first child. Zorn began a study of the subject, reading medical journals and attending workshops, and had a successful VBAC with her second child, born in 1981.

Convinced that there was a need for a central headquarters, a clearinghouse of up-to-date information and exchange of views for women in a similar predicament, Zorn decided to publish a newsletter, *The Clarion*. She sent the first issue, dated June 1982, to five hundred women across the country. Within two months she had to reprint it, the demand having quickly spread by word of mouth.

By 1991 the Cesarean Prevention Movement had seventy-two chapters in thirty states, twelve in California alone.* *The Clarion* has a circulation of ten thousand.

The explicit goals of CPM are threefold: 'to lower the rising Caesarean rate through education; to provide a forum where women and men can express their concerns about birth; and to provide a support network for women who are healing from past birth experiences and those who are preparing for future births.'

CPM is not a home-birth organisation, nor does it refer mothers to specific doctors or midwives; the idea is to encourage women to make their own decisions and to inform them about their choices. Although there was resistance in medical circles, some physicians

* In 1992 the name was changed to Cesarean Awareness Movement.

have themselves started CPM chapters, recognising the importance to women of sharing ideas, and of mutual support.

Esther Zorn, a level-headed type who by no means opposes all Caesareans but recognises the need in many life-threatening situations, is mainly intent on providing basic consumer education to pregnant women: 'We know more about the microwave ovens we buy than about the hospital services we purchase for our unborn children!' She cites the Maternity Information Act in Massachusetts*, which requires hospitals to disclose Caesarean rates and other information, such as use of epidurals, induction of labour, and VBACs.

While get-togethers at which women who belong to the Cesarean Prevention Movement discuss their feelings of disappointment or outrage about their Caesareans may have therapeutic value, there is an occasional distressing tendency to wallow in self-pity, as in this hyperbolic description by a mother in a CPM newsletter. Although by her own account the Caesarean was necessary in the circumstances, she writes: 'They come, thieves with knives. I will be shut out, a passive, inert body to be cut open, my baby stolen from my uterus . . . They don't even know what is lost is so dear, they don't see the rape, the theft, the violation of my body . . .' and lots more rich, beautiful prose along the same lines.

A bracingly different perspective was offered by Linda Kalman of Rancho Palos Verdes in Southern California. An accomplished horsewoman who regularly exhibits in horse shows, she was twenty-nine in 1982 when she became pregnant with her first child. With her doctor's agreement, she continued to ride and compete in horse shows until the seventh month, when these activities became too uncomfortable.

About two and a half weeks beyond her due date, she went to the hospital with contractions that lasted for several hours – 'no dilation, just progressively sharper pains. All in all, the prebirth experience was one of the most painful events of my life, including breaking a leg, concussions, et cetera, and I was grateful for the opportunity for the C-section.'

The doctor said the foetal monitor showed that the baby was

* Passed on December 31, 1985.

under stress, and he suggested a C-section; 'I was all too glad to be finally done with this job. I asked for a general anaesthetic and my little girl was eventually born around six-thirty a.m.'

Ms Kalman says she doesn't remember experiencing much post-operative pain: 'I was so high from the birth of my little girl it wouldn't have mattered anyway.'

As one might have guessed from the foregoing, the day after surgery this stalwart Amazon was 'parading up and down the hospital halls' carrying her baby and nursing her. Four weeks after she returned home she started riding again, and at five weeks rode her horse in a show – 'bouncy breasts and all!' as she told me.

Two years later her son, Christopher, was born, again about three weeks overdue; after some deliberation, at her doctor's advice she had another C-section. Her reflections on the subject:

'If I was to become pregnant again, I might try to have a natural birth, just for the experience, but I don't have strong feelings one way or the other. As far as I am concerned, the important part is what happens after the baby comes out – how he/she gets out is really irrelevant, I believe. I love both my kids dearly. How they came into being really seems beside the point – it was a long time ago, the memories are fading, and who cares anyway? They are here now, and they are both wonderful.'

Once again, iatrogenesis – or illness caused by doctors – rears its ugly head. In a paper titled 'The Relationship of Obstetrical Trauma to Learning Disabilities: An Obstetrician's View', Don Creevy of the Stanford University School of Medicine has written, 'If there is a causal relationship between certain perinatal events and learning disabilities, it follows that if a physician causes such a perinatal event, he or she has increased the probability of occurrence of the learning disability. An obvious example is the case of an ill-planned induction of labour or elective repeat Caesarean in which the baby turns out to be premature. The physician, by causing the baby to be born prematurely, has subjected the baby to an increased risk of all kinds of problems, including learning disabilities.'

Estimates of maternal deaths subsequent to Caesareans vary considerably. Mortimer Rosen found that the maternal mortality rate for Caesarean mothers is four times as high – 41 per 100,000 births – as for those delivered vaginally; and even for a scheduled Caesarean (as distinct from an emergency), a woman is twice as likely to die as a woman going through vaginal birth. Creevy referred to 'the known fact that maternal mortality is increased from two to thirty times by C-section', citing a study on Caesarean section and maternal mortality in Rhode Island.

The Institute of Medicine has thrown in the towel, observing that 'the studies comparing maternal mortality from vaginal and cesarean deliveries are in conflict' and adding, 'All studies show that Caesarean section delivery does increase maternal morbidity, including increased incidence of infection, longer hospitalisation, problems of bonding with the infant, as well as rarer complications, including hysterectomy and bowel trauma.'

Books and articles of advice to the pregnant woman on how to choose an obstetrician frequently stress the importance of ascertaining the doctor's Caesarean rate. This may be easier said than done, for within the profession the rates for individual practitioners are often a closely held secret; or the physician may not in fact know her/his own rate, or may claim not to know. As the head of the nursing programme in a California community college told me, 'The doctor's lawyer might tell him such records should not be available for subpoena. They just don't keep the data because it may be damaging in court, and they want to protect themselves.'

According to the Public Citizen Health Research Group, whose researchers conducted a vast, nationwide, state-by-state, hospital-by-hospital survey on all aspects of the Caesarean controversy: 'Rates for individual physicians were only available from Maryland for this study. The availability of information on the practice of individual physicians has been a controversial issue, with medical societies vigorously opposing the availability of this important information. In Maryland, physicians' names were not available, but simply a code number.' A close look at the code numbers revealed a wide range of Caesarean rates in 1987 for Maryland practitioners – from 0 per cent to 57 per cent, with a mean of 27 per cent – but the hapless Maryland woman seeking information about individual practitioners would have no way of discovering who's who in this numerical thicket.

Even more alarming is the atmosphere of secrecy surrounding 'peer review' sessions, in which hospital staff discuss and analyse the treatment of individual cases. In a teaching hospital, medical students normally attend these meetings as part of their obstetrical training. The committee charged by the Institute of Medicine with examining the effects of malpractice insurance on the practice of obstetrics found that rules and regulations had been revised to forbid participation of medical students and other health professionals in such meetings: 'One respondent reported that, as a response to the current professional liability climate, "We have closed our Morbidity and Mortality Teaching Conference to students, nurses, and other ancillary personnel who may not understand or may misinterpret the frank criticism of management of specific cases." Thus, it appears that, in the view of many respondents, the medical liability climate is also undermining the teaching and training of medical students.'

Visualised in terms of a stage drama, the three principal performers in a hospital birth scene are the doctor, the patient, and her unborn child. Walk-on parts include nurses, anaesthetists, and other hospital personnel; waiting in the wings are the baby's father and other family friends, if present. It goes without saying that none of these bit players would be consulted as to the advisability, in any given case, of a Caesarean; or such has been the experience of many women with whom I have discussed the matter. However, this must vary from hospital to hospital. Dr Rhoda Nussbaum at Kaiser Permanente in San Francisco disputed the notion that the family would not be participants and would not be fully informed of all details ahead of surgery. 'In Kaiser, the "bit players" certainly *are* involved,' she said.

But in the last analysis the physician in charge is alone empowered, after consultation with other obstetricians, to decide on a Caesarean, based on various criteria – the most important of which is (or should be) the medical diagnosis, the paramount concern for the safety of mother and child. Too often the medical decision may be distorted by misinterpretation of the foetal electronic monitor tracing; inability to use forceps or vacuum extractor due to lack of training or experience; or a simple lack of know-how in managing vaginal breech delivery.

Aside from the welfare of mother and baby, there are other considerations, less altruistic: profitability for doctor and hospital; convenience for doctor – and sometimes ditto for mother; overriding – the looming spectre of malpractice suits.

To discuss these in turn:

MEDICAL DIAGNOSES

Medical indications for a Caesarean include maternal illness such as diabetes, high blood pressure, and active genital herpes (which could infect the baby in its passage through the birth canal); haemorrhage from the uterus, potentially dangerous for both mother and child; prolapsed cord, meaning the umbilical cord is beside or ahead of the unborn baby, cutting off its oxygen supply; and 'transverse lie', meaning that the baby is lying sideways across the mother's abdomen, rendering normal delivery impossible.

Further reasons for the operation that are considered medically valid by mainstream obstetricians, although strongly contested by other medical practitioners, including physicians and experienced midwives, are twin or multiple births, and 'breech birth', meaning that the baby is in the wrong position – feet first or buttocks first. Even assuming (the dissenters say) that every effort at 'version', turning the baby by manual manipulation through the mother's abdomen, may have failed, vaginal delivery of these balky babes can still be satisfactorily accomplished, given patience on the part of the birth attendants and cooperation by the mother.

In the fairly extensive realm of medical obfuscation are three catch-all diagnoses that together account for at least 38 per cent of primary Caesareans: cephalopelvic disproportion, dystocia, and foetal distress. One can imagine the apprehension of a young woman in labour, strapped into her electronic monitor, as the doctor peers down at her and announces in gloomy tones that she is suffering from dystocia. 'Would you please explain what that means?' she might ask; or, depending on her mood of the moment, 'What the hell is that?'

Dystocia is doctor language for a poor fit between mother and baby, making normal delivery difficult or impossible. This would be the case if the mother had a deformed pelvis due to disease, such as polio – common 40 years ago, now extremely rare. Today, dystocia may be suspected if the doctor thinks the baby is too big, the mother's pelvis too small; but this cannot be predicted with any accuracy, as the pelvis, an irregular passageway of bone and muscle, has its own way of reacting to the oncoming baby. The doctor can almost never tell by a vaginal examination that a pelvis is too small for a normal birth. But clearly, in the rare situations where real dystocia means that vaginal birth is impossible, Caesarean delivery is one of those truly lifesaving medical innovations that one can but applaud.

The textbook definition of dystocia is 'difficult labour due to mechanical factors produced by the foetus or the maternal pelvis, or due to inadequate uterine or other muscular activity.'

The trouble arose when doctors started expanding the definition of dystocia to cover a multitude of conditions, summed up specifically as 'failure to progress' in labour, a purely subjective judgment that varies from doctor to doctor. As described by Dr Mortimer Rosen, one physician may make the diagnosis after six or eight hours and go to a Caesarean; another may wait eighteen hours before operating; yet another may wait twenty-four hours and do a successful vaginal delivery. 'For most doctors,' Dr Rosen has written, 'dystocia now means, "This baby should have been born by now and I don't know why it hasn't."'

An eminently plausible answer to that question is that 'failure to progress' is likely to be iatrogenic in origin, meaning an illness or dangerous physical condition caused by the ministrations of the *soi-disant* practitioners of the healing arts. Epidurals and other anaesthetics can be a potent factor in slowing down, or even stopping, labour. The situation of a woman lying flat on her back, with the electronic foetal monitor strapped on to her, denied food and drink, unable to walk about at will, confined in the unfamiliar setting of a hospital labour room, is a considerable hindrance to progress in labour. She might not even have the reassuring presence of a solicitous nurse, as the nurse will be busy in another room reading the EFM printouts.

What precisely is meant by normal progress of labour? A further indication for a Caesarean may arise from reliance by the physician on the Friedman Curve. This purports to divulge to a compliant medical profession the correct amount of time that should be allowed for each stage of labour. (Do I hear Voices Off, in tones of admiration or derision, chorusing, 'Only a man could have thought *that* up!'?)

Emanuel Friedman of Harvard Medical School, using data from deliveries by a large number of women, charted the average time from start to finish of the three stages of labour and in 1978 evolved what he regarded as definitive answers. For example, he concluded that the 'Latent Phase' of the First Stage of labour, in which contractions are quite far apart and the cervical dilation is progressing slowly from 2 to 4 centimetres, should take 8.6 hours. Next, speeding up rather quickly, is the 'Active Phase' of the First Stage of labour, shown as a steep rise on Friedman's graph. In this phase, dilation goes to 8 centimetres. Then the rate of acceleration decreases until the cervix is opened to its maximum of 10 centimetres. Friedman said this deceleration phase, which completes the First Stage, should not exceed three hours for a woman labouring with her firstborn, and one hour for subsequent babies.

The Second Stage, from full dilation of the cervix to expulsion of the infant, he said, should be completed in one hour for a first birth and fifteen minutes for subsequent births, by the end of which the baby should be born. (The Third Stage is the expulsion of the placenta.)

It may have been an enjoyable moment for Friedman when, having got all his facts and figures in order, he at last reached the stage of entering them on a chart to be printed and disseminated to maternity wards throughout the nation. It must be a lot less fun for the prospective mother, striving for the finish line like an Olympic Games contestant, hoping against hope that her case will fall within the 'normal' limits. Her own individual graph, based on the Friedman principles, will be prepared by the nursing staff.

Of all the fads and fancies adopted by the medical profession in the era of high technology, the Friedman Curve must rank as one of the weirdest and most out of touch with reality. As most mothers can affirm – especially those who have had several children – it is well nigh impossible to pinpoint with any accuracy just when the 'Latent Phase', or first-stage labour, contractions began. For some, mild contractions can continue for several days – and still be perfectly normal – before the woman decides it's time to go to the hospital. What, then, becomes of her 8.6-hour deadline? Worse yet, should she exceed Dr Friedman's allotted time of 2.5 hours for 'Active Phase', or second-stage labour, she may be found guilty of 'failure to progress'.

Commenting on the Friedman Curve, the National Institutes of Health have observed, 'The concept that slow progress constitutes abnormal progress permeates current obstetrical thinking . . . Thus, delivery for all patients in less than 24 hours has been advocated, as has intervention after two to four hours of poor progress in active labor.'

The whole concept of a preordained average time for the various stages of labour, from which one deviates at one's peril, is absurd to trained midwives, who know from experience that there is no 'norm', each case presenting its own specific peculiarities of timing in which artificial deadlines have no place – are, in fact, worse than meaningless.

As for 'foetal distress', that requires no elaborate explanation; the woman sweating and straining away in the delivery room knows exactly what it means: her baby is in mortal danger. Is it, or isn't it? Again, this depends entirely on the individual judgment of the doctor in charge.

Real foetal distress can indeed be fatal, resulting in a stillborn or a dying newborn, or a survivor who may be hopelessly brain-damaged. The main cause is lack of oxygen – for example if the umbilical cord is too short and wound tightly around the unborn baby's neck, cutting off its oxygen supply (one-fourth to one-third are born with the cord around the neck and are not affected at all); or a lethal condition called placenta previa, meaning that the placenta, or afterbirth, comes ahead of the baby and blocks it off from freedom and fresh air. Such conditions, in which a Caesarean is the only known way to deliver the baby successfully, are fortunately extremely rare, about 1 in 250 cases.

Much less rare is the diagnosis of 'foetal distress' where it may not in fact exist. According to the Public Citizen Health Research Group, undue reliance on the electronic foetal monitor is the principal reason for the overprediction of foetal distress, known as 'false positives'. The group has cited a German study which found that for every infant with real foetal distress, both in high- and low-risk groups, three infants showed false signs of distress. Thus if physicians relied exclusively on EFM to decide whether to perform a Caesarean, three women would have unnecessary Caesareans for every infant with real foetal distress.

In their examination of hospital records, the researchers discovered that in Maryland in 1987 the diagnosis of foetal distress varied greatly from hospital to hospital – from a low of three per cent to a high of 30 per cent. 'There is no medical reason that would explain why there is over a tenfold difference in the rate of foetal distress from one hospital to another,' they concluded. 'At this point, the diagnosis of foetal distress becomes absolutely meaningless.'

Dr Greg Troll, whose early career as a lay midwife was a potent factor in shaping his philosophy about birth, admitted that his years of medical training caused him to modify somewhat his opinions.

'I'm still a little schizophrenic,' he said. 'I have midwife instinct, and I try not to pull the doctor out of the closet unless he's needed, but he's always there. I still feel that things aren't going to go wrong, but boy, I know what *can* go wrong very, very well.'

A case in point is the often agonising decision whether or not to do a Caesarean – 'It's major surgery, no doubt about it,' Greg said. 'It involves risks of anaesthesia, risks of haemorrhage, risks of blood replacement. I'm one hundred per cent into Caesarean prevention, but when you can't prevent it I think Caesarean is a wonderful procedure. I learned to feel comfortable with a C-section despite my bias against it.

'Once you go into the operating room you have this great feeling of relief. It's really interesting – I'm talking about the doctor now, not the patient, right? She's not progressing, she's complaining. Her family is on my case, they're demanding that we operate. I urge patience, let her labour longer, let's give her more support. But once I've caved in, and said, "All right, we'll go to a Caesarean" – *whew!* Now I'm in control, I've got a clear field. I've got anaesthesia, I call in my consultant, I know exactly how to proceed. Going to the operating room was very stress-reducing for me.'

I asked Greg whether, in view of the fact that in many advanced European countries medical experts consider a rate of five to seven per cent Caesareans to be the norm, the Natividad Medical Center in Salinas rate of 17 to 19 per cent wasn't rather high? 'A five per cent rate or lower can be totally reasonable if the women are well fed, well educated, and well supported in labour,' he said, 'and you have an attentive staff who know what true signs of trouble are as opposed to a funny thing on a foetal monitor artifact that everybody overreacts to because they're tired. The Caesarean rate has gone way up because of electronic foetal monitoring.'

For a further opinion on the advantages and disadvantages of the inexorable march forward of medical science as it affects the birth scene, I consulted Jennifer Dohrn, whose pioneering work at the Childbearing Center of Morris Heights will be described in Chapter 13.

Like Greg Troll, Dohrn is a midwife by training and philosophical outlook, and an implacable opponent of high-tech procedures routinely adhered to in American maternity wards. Speaking to me in 1991 about the obvious benefits of advanced techniques, invaluable in specific rare cases, she sounded a note of frustration:

> What's so incredibly tragic and ironic is the fact that with modern technology, when there are complications, we can have a very high rate of healthy mothers and babies by using techniques that have been developed to deal with complications. The problem is, of course, that this is being used without discretion. It's being used across the board, many levels of intervention, and women are placed in situations that are frightening and disrespectful and expected to have, quote, 'normal' labours and births.

In the 1980s, Ms Dohrn worked for some years in Nicaragua helping the Sandinistas 'build a different kind of health care system, progressive and humane and revolutionary in the true sense'. It was there, in the mountainous region of Matagalpa, that the paradox of the high-tech controversy came home to her. About fifty *parteras*, lay midwives from different rural communities, had hiked along mountain trails to meet a group of American midwives to discuss all aspects of birth from prenatal to delivery to postnatal care.

And as the discussion got very animated, I remember one *partera* jumping up and saying, 'Now you can tell us, now you can tell us what you do. What do you do when the placenta comes first?' And there was this awful moment of silence among the American midwives, because the placenta coming first, a condition known as placenta previa, is life-threatening to mother and baby and without an immediate Caesarean section, certainly the baby and probably the mother will die. And our response, of course, is we go to the hospital, and they were in the situation where there was no hospital to go to, and it meant certain death of the infant and possibly haemorrhaging to death of the mother.

Warming to the theme, Ms Dohrn continued:

It's circumstances like this that make me respectful of the potential that we have for truly changing health care because of the level of technology in this country, and also makes me extremely angry about how it's so grossly misused. So instead of it being our friend, and having it there when we need it, it is used in what to me is a grossly incorrect way for women and families in this country.

COD AND ASAP

These well-known abbreviations for 'cash on delivery' and 'as soon as possible' might seem, to the average well-informed Doubting Thomases (or more likely Thomasinas), to sum up what they already instinctively knew: that doctors and hospitals make huge profits out of Caesareans, of which, it turns out, the majority are unnecessary; and that these are timed for the convenience of the doctor.

To dispose of the ASAP factor: as far as I know, there have been no research studies on this, no massive surveys to discover when the astrological signs are most propitious for a Caesarean. My findings are purely anecdotal, from discussions around the States with hospital personnel involved in the process on a day-to-day basis. The 'elective' Caesarean, as distinct from the real or perceived emergency decided on at the last minute, is extremely convenient for the doctor, as he can schedule the operation whenever it suits him; he doesn't have to hang around waiting for the mother to deliver vaginally. (Actually he doesn't hang about much anyway, but mostly shows up at the last minute, if then. You can ask anyone who has with great forethought chosen the best doctor she can find; too often, the actual event will be attended by a stand-in whom she has never set eyes on before.)

Prime time for Caesareans is before 5:30 p.m., which won't interfere with Doctor's dinner hour. I have been told by a lawyer who made a study of this phenomenon that just before major holidays – Christmas, New Year's Eve, Thanksgiving – the C-section rate of some doctors soars above 75 per cent, three times the national average. It must be said that for some mothers the prearranged elective Caesarean can also be something of a boon, enabling them to arrange their social schedule accordingly. According to Dr Warren Pearse of the American College of Obstetricians and Gynecologists, in Brazil for that very reason, Caesarean is the preference of rich society women and accounts for 90 per cent of private clinic births in that country. Dr Patricia Macnair, writing in the London *Independent*, elaborates: 'Would you like to keep your vagina "honeymoon fresh?" This suggestion, made regularly in Brazil to encourage pregnant women to have a Caesarean delivery is among several factors that contribute to one of the highest Caesarean birth rates in the world.'

Now for the COD aspect. The Public Citizen Health Research Group estimated that unnecessary Caesareans accounted annually for an extra 1.1 million days in the hospital and cost over $1 billion. Of more interest are the whys and wherefores of physician-mandated Caesareans.

Jane Brody in *The New York Times* put it rather bluntly, saying:

> a common accusation is that greed is responsible for the rising rate of Caesareans. Doctors usually earn 20 to 40 percent more and hospitals may double their revenue with a Caesarean birth. This is difficult to prove, of course, but critics note that Caesarean rate is highest in private hospitals and lowest in municipal hospitals. They also note that resident physicians, who are salaried, are much less likely to operate than private obstetricians, who receive a fee for services.

One of the more ambitious efforts to determine whether there was a correlation between income and Caesarean rates was undertaken by Dr Jeffrey B. Gould and colleagues, as reported in the *New England Journal of Medicine*. They painstakingly sorted through birth-certificate data for 245,854 births in Los Angeles County in 1982 and 1983, and then broke these down by census tracts showing median family income. Their findings: independent of maternal age, parity, or birth weight, women who lived in census tracts with a median family income of $30,000 had a primary C-section rate of 22.9 per cent, compared with a rate of 13.2 per cent for women from areas with a median family income of under $11,000.

Searching for possible reasons for the disparity, Gould et al. noted:

> The observed differences may reflect the different settings in which the rich and poor receive their obstetrical care. The poor are more likely to give birth in public hospitals and have their health care costs covered by Medicaid, and they are less likely to have private physicians. Alternatively, different clinical decision-making rules may be applied to poor women, regardless of differences in the health care setting. For instance, it may be that the greater social congruity between obstetricians and middle-class parturients leads to differences in clinical management.

Or, to paraphrase F. Scott Fitzgerald's legendary colloquy with Ernest Hemingway: 'The rich are different from you and me.' 'Yes they have more cesareans.'

Dr Gould was himself puzzled at the outcome of his study. He told the press, 'The most surprising thing is that one expects poor people to have many more health problems than rich people. They have more low-birth-weight babies and more mortality. The notion that rich people are having more cesarean sections than poor people is a topsy-turvy finding.' Asked why this should be, he suspected that doctors might be quicker to do a Caesarean on affluent women, because of the fear that these patients are more likely to sue if their babies have problems during vaginal births.

Following up on the report by the Public Citizen Health Research Group, some metropolitan dailies highlighted its findings as related to their own communities. The *Atlanta Journal & Constitution* featured a chart showing the Caesarean rates in several for-profit hospitals ranging from 42.5 per cent to 32.6 per cent, whereas Grady Memorial Hospital in Atlanta, which delivers babies to more indigent mothers than any other hospital in the state, had one of Georgia's lowest rates – 18.7 per cent.

Peter Aleshire, author of 'Science Watch' in the Oakland (California) *Tribune*, reviewing C-section rates in various hospitals in the area, noted that 'at the top of the list we find some of the hospitals best known in the medical community for their devotion to business'. Six of these, all catering to privately insured patients, have rates from 33 to 38 per cent. At the bottom end of the list are the Kaiser hospitals and the county hospitals. Since doctors there work for the hospitals, and patients don't pay itemised bills, neither doctor nor hospital collects more money for C-sections.

MALPRACTICE INSURANCE: THE DOCTOR'S DILEMMA
(and even more, come to think of it, the Patient's Dilemma)

What is known in medical circles as the 'malpractice insurance crisis', meaning the skyrocketing cost of such insurance, began in the mid-1970s and escalated throughout the 1980s, with no end in sight for the 1990s. The alarming rise in malpractice premiums, most notably in the practice of obstetrics, has caused widespread abandonment by obstetricians of their specialty, as well as a parallel flight from the birth scene of general practitioners and family doctors who, if they include delivery of babies in their practice, must pay approximately twice their regular annual premium.

In consequence, there are vast areas of the country – particularly in rural communities – where no obstetrical services whatsoever are available to the pregnant woman. For poor women in both town and country there are, as we have seen in Chapter 4, almost insurmountable roadblocks to getting prenatal care, and scant chance of getting decent treatment should they arrive in labour in some overcrowded hospital emergency room. Accounts of babies being born unattended in hospital corridors abound in medical circles. Experts in high places deplore this state of affairs; as Warren Pearse of the American College of Obstetricians and Gynecologists told me in April 1990, 'Today, access to obstetric care is a major problem for women in this country. Too many persons who want obstetrical care simply cannot find it.' And again: 'We have overwhelming problems with access to maternity care today.'

The astronomic rise in malpractice insurance premiums is ascribed variously by the medical community to the general litigiousness of American society, the rapacity of personal-injury lawyers with their wily ways of persuading juries to award outlandish damages, and the publicity given to such huge awards, which encourage further lawsuits against doctors by dissatisfied patients.

But from the patient's point of view, living in a nation which alone among industrialised countries (with the exception of South Africa) has no national health service and makes no provision for the care of a citizen who may have suffered a lifelong injury at the hands of an incompetent doctor, a lawsuit may well seem the only logical route. And for a mother whose baby was born with irreversible brain damage because of medical ineptitude, a verdict in the millions of dollars would by no means seem excessive, given the computed cost of its care for life.

The cost of malpractice insurance varies greatly among medical specialties and also from state to state. For the specialists, at the bottom rung are the dermatologists; although they may charge a fortune for treating teenage acne (for which until recently there was no known cure, except the passage of time), they are unlikely to do much serious harm. Close to the top are neurosurgeons, orthopaedists, and thoracic surgeons. At the pinnacle are obstetricians.

A few pointers along the road, supplied by researchers for the American College of Obstetricians and Gynecologists – to which about 95 per cent of practitioners in those specialties belong:

The national average malpractice premium for obstetricians in 1989 was 348 per cent higher than it had been in 1983, having risen from $10,946 to $38,138.

ACOG's latest survey, released on September 12, 1990, showed that 77.6 per cent of obstetricians had at least one claim filed against them, up from 70.6 per cent in the 1987 survey. Of these, 18 per cent had been sued twice, 13 per cent three times, and 23 per cent four times.

ACOG's profile of the typical OB/GYN practitioner: forty-seven years old, has been in practice sixteen years, has experienced *three* malpractice suits, up from an average of 1.7 in 1987. Of those claims, 31.4 per cent were for brain damage suffered by the new-born.

A complete state-by-state listing in ACOG's 1990 fact sheet shows a huge disparity in annual premiums paid by obstetricians. 'Rates vary depending on the legal system and climate within the state,' Dr Pearse told me, and indeed they do: all the way from Florida, at the top with a premium of $202,800, to Arkansas, at the bottom with $20,000. In between are rich states like New York, $106,600; and poor states like South Dakota, $23,500, and South Carolina, $23,600.

However, reading on through the ACOG material, it appears that things are not as gloomy for the doctors as they might seem at first blush:

Almost 40 per cent of all claims were dropped or settled without payment.

OB/GYNs won 68.6 per cent of the claims that went to arbitration or to a jury.

The average amount paid on obstetrician claims was $311,378. For a brain-damaged infant: $597,000.

These are a far cry from the multimillion-dollar verdicts that appear in the papers; but one should bear in mind that such awards are often drastically reduced by the trial judge, news that generally goes unreported; and that the plaintiff's legal fees will eat up a third to a half of the amount awarded.

In its two-volume 1989 survey of the medical malpractice scene, the Institute of Medicine has noted that 'despite the fact that jury verdicts in medical malpractice cases are roundly criticized, there have been surprisingly few studies of what actually happens in mal-practice cases that go to court, and virtually no studies of cases involving obstetricians and gynecologists . . . The accepted wisdom blames the legal system for the problems faced by doctors. Physicians have argued that there are too many lawsuits, too many jury awards for plaintiffs . . . In contrast, we find that few of these cases go before a jury, that plaintiffs do not usually win.'

The report states that on average one in twenty hospital patients suffers injury as a result of medical errors. (The report is not referring here only to obstetrical cases, nor to instances of significant and permanent injury; just to mishaps, large and small, that occur in hospitals.) Few instances of injury caused by doctors lead to an insurance claim: 'At most, one in ten such injuries resulted in a claim, and of those only 40 percent received payment. At most, one in 25 negligent injuries results in compensation via the malpractice system.'

Why so few lawsuits for malpractice? For one thing, a patient can easily be misled by the doctor and hospital staff as to the cause of his or her injury. Unfamiliar with medical terminology, he or she may be sweet-talked into the belief that whatever went wrong was certainly not the fault of anybody connected with treatment of the malady. Furthermore, lawyers are very reluctant to get involved in malpractice cases. The big-time ambulance chasers are far happier with those spectacular flaming plane crashes with multiple deaths and injuries, in which everyone can be sued from the airline company to the plane manufacturer – all multibillion-dollar corporations. In comparison, malpractice cases are on the whole very small potatoes and extremely hard to prove in court, which accounts for the large number of out-of-court settlements. An obvious prerequisite is convincing medical testimony by a reputable physician; but doctors are notoriously reluctant to testify for the plaintiff against one of their own. The profession has its own ways of punishing those who do testify.

There is, however, another side to it. As an internist and public-health specialist – who is a strong consumer advocate – pointed out to me, by no means *all* abnormal obstetrical outcomes – brain damage, etc. – are the result of malpractice or incompetence; and neither are all malpractice suits justified.

'Despite good care and accepted practice, whether by doctor or midwife, every once in a while things go wrong, and the baby is damaged,' he said. 'One can understand how a family feels it must be all the doctor's fault since there was no forewarning of the abnormal outcome. And the plaintiff's lawyer asks: Did the doctor do absolutely *everything* to prevent the injury? Hence the predictable increase in the use of EFM and Caesareans – directly traceable to the threat of malpractice litigation.'

To get a trial lawyer's perspective on this, I sought out several who specialise in malpractice litigation. How difficult is it to get a physician to testify against another? What is the cost of bringing such a lawsuit? Is America, as widely perceived, a peculiarly litigious society? Some comments:

Stephen Cooper of Los Angeles, who has tried numerous cases in Southern California, said that there are doctors in that area willing to testify – 'but if the defendant obstetrician is a popular, well-known personage in the community it might be necessary to get an out-of-state expert witness'.

Attorney Janice Wezelman of Tucson, Arizona, in 1990 won a spectacular, highly newsworthy jury verdict of $4.25 million for a brain-damaged child born in 1978. The case dragged on for twelve years, Ms Wezelman taking over in 1988 from a former colleague in her law firm. The injured child, twelve years old as of this writing, has the IQ of a two-year-old. How did Ms Wezelman's law firm happen to get the case? 'The mother, a poor woman, a patient in the county hospital, was probably advised by a family friend to get a lawyer.' As to general litigiousness, Ms Wezelman referred to articles in the *New England Journal of Medicine* of February 7, 1991, and July 23, 1991: 'They concluded that for every sixty-five hundred people who are hospitalised sixty-five will be injured through negligence, but only one of those sixty-five will file a lawsuit.'

James Bostwick, a San Francisco lawyer whose practice, he told me, is 'one hundred per cent plaintiffs' personal-injury cases,' is known nationally for his expertise in lawsuits involving childbirth. He has tried at least two hundred of these over the years, ranging from haemorrhage by the mother to the death of or permanent damage to the newborn.

Mr Bostwick's largest damage award for a brain-damaged baby was $3.6 million, in a case against a county hospital in the early 1980s. 'That might not sound like much, but since 1975 California law only allows two hundred fifty thousand dollars for "pain and suffering",' he said. The mother, a county patient, had asked for a Caesarean, as she had had a pelvic fracture. In a switch from the picture of the knife-happy obstetrician, this doctor refused the Caesarean. 'It's a macho thing,' Mr Bostwick said. 'They want to prove they can do a vaginal birth, so they tell the woman who wants a Caesarean, "No." During labour everything went wrong. There was a failed attempt to deliver with forceps. When it was born, the child didn't breathe for an hour. Before trial, the electronic foetal monitor records were "lost".'

Is it difficult to get doctors to testify against their colleagues? I asked Bostwick. 'It was virtually impossible in the late 1960s and early '70s. But by the mid-1970s it became fashionable in medical circles to recognise a social responsibility that might require them to appear in court on behalf of a damaged victim of malpractice. Also, they charge huge fees – five hundred dollars an hour for consultation, five thousand dollars a day to testify in court. In contrast, the highest per-hour charge by lawyers is three hundred dollars, but that's exceptional; most charge about one hundred twenty-five to one hundred fifty dollars.' Even today, when doctors are more amenable to testifying, they run a risk. 'They can still be blackballed – even professors in universities; colleagues may come down on them. Obstetricians may face a boycott – refusal of other OBs to refer cases, revocation of hospital privileges.

'Of the whole spectrum of personal-injury cases those involving childbirth are the most difficult, the most expensive, and the hardest to win,' Bostwick said. 'It costs at least one hundred thousand dollars to prepare a case. You may have to go from California to Boston for an expert willing to testify, then fly him to San Francisco for depositions and trial.' Under the contingent fee arrangement, these costs are assumed by the lawyer, recoverable only if and when he or she settles the case or gets a jury award for the client.

As to the much-touted litigiousness of Americans, Bostwick thinks the opposite is true: 'Most people don't like litigation; they only go that route when they've got no choice. Among the most litigious are professional people, especially doctors!'

*

There is across-the-board agreement that fear of being sued has had a dramatic effect on the day-to-day practice of medicine in general and obstetrics in particular. Sophisticated ultra-modern diagnostic devices, formerly used only when the doctor suspected some serious complication, are now called into service as part of every routine check-up – provided, however, that the cost of the tests is recoverable from the patient's private insurance or from Medicaid.

In the area of childbirth, as the 1989 Institute of Medicine report put it, 'There is no question that physicians themselves firmly believe that the current medical liability climate has prompted them to change the way in which they practice obstetrics. According to the American College of Obstetricians and Gynecologists (1985), 41 percent of obstetricians said they have altered the way they practice as a result of the risk of medical liability.' Foremost among the changes: 'increased use of testing and other diagnostic and monitoring procedures'.

The report made some acerbic comments on the almost universal acceptance of electronic foetal monitors by the obstetrical community – despite the fact that the monitors have 'never been formally evaluated by the Food and Drug Administration' or by the Department of Health and Human Services, both charged by law with overseeing the use of new devices. Furthermore, 'third-party insurers such as Blue Cross and Medicaid, which are in a position to evaluate new procedures, failed to question the efficacy of EFM before setting their reimbursement rates for the procedure.' Hence third-party payment for EFM is readily available via major insurance programmes or via Medicaid, which generally follows the major insurers' lead.

The inevitable chain of events arising from electronic foetal monitoring was summarised in the report, which concluded that the current professional liability climate supports the continued use of EFM despite 'overwhelming evidence that it does not improve neonatal mortality and morbidity rates'. Foetal heart rate tracings are likely to be overread, over-cautiously interpreted, leading to more Caesareans; foetal monitoring by itself will increase the rate of intervention; there is a higher incidence of dystocia among women who have continuous EFM, as they are unable to walk around and are therefore less able to tolerate labour and require more sedation.

And finally, 'There is overwhelming evidence that part of the recent rise in the Cesarean section rate in this country is the result of the medical-legal environment. Given the current siege mentality among clinicians, one wonders why the Cesarean rate is not higher.'

From the obstetrician's point of view, the EFM printout with its dramatic ups and downs showing all manner of bad possibilities for the unborn baby – and never mind that these have been proved to be inefficient indicators – can be the key to successful defence should he become a defendant in a lawsuit.

He may have in mind the ancient proverb 'For want of a shoe the horse was lost; for want of a horse the rider was lost; for want of a rider the battle was lost . . .' Translated into modern obstetrical terms, the moral might emerge that 'For want of an electronic foetal monitor, the printout was lost; for want of a printout, the evidence was lost; for want of a Caesarean, the lawsuit was lost.'

PART FOUR

Midwives

Chapter 9

IN SEARCH OF MIDWIVES

In *The Lancet* of October 9, 1847, W. Tyler Smith, M.B. (Bachelor of Medicine) set forth his views about midwives. 'Modern obstetric practice has gradually advanced,' he wrote, 'to be acknowledged as one of the three primary departments of medicine.' He continued:

In this country the midwife is very much out of date, belonging to a bygone, rather than to the present age. The great mass of our obstetric practice is a ministration of education and experience, such as no endeavours could impart to a body of females . . .

I think the progress of this branch of our art will hereafter demand that the office of the midwife be abolished altogether . . .

It should be the steady aim of every man engaged in obstetric practice . . . to discourage midwife practice . . . This department of the profession will never take its true rank until this reform has been effected.

On the whole, Dr Smith's words of wisdom fell on deaf ears in most of Europe, where to this day midwives are the principal birth attendants and are, according to the World Health Organization, largely responsible for the low incidence of infant deaths in those countries where their services are most often employed.

But in America, organised medicine has been largely successful in driving midwives from the birth scene. In 1900, about 50 per cent of American births were attended by midwives; by 1935 the rate had fallen to 12 per cent, and most of those were in the black population of the Deep South. By 1986, only about four per cent of pregnant women were getting nurse-midwife care.

For a briefing on the general status, worldwide, of midwives, I arranged to meet Sheila Kitzinger, something of a legend in her own time, in London. Jon Snow, newscaster with Channel 4 put it succinctly: 'To English people of my generation, in their thirties and forties, Sheila Kitzinger is as famous as Dr Spock would be to Americans of your age.' She has published more than twenty acclaimed books on birth-related subjects; has had an enormous influence on the natural childbirth/home birth trend; has been the subject of innumerable articles in the popular press; and is in demand for television interviews. She travels around the world lecturing and exhorting on her subject. In short, she is a founding mother of the back-to-nature, forward-to-unmedicated-home-birth movement.

At the time of our meeting, in the autumn of 1989, I was staying with the writer Sally Belfrage, daughter of Cedric Belfrage and, in fact, the skinned rabbit named Fred that figured in Cedric's long-ago account of her birth under Twilight Sleep. As Sheila Kitzinger was coming all the way from the Cotswolds by train, we thought she would be very hungry, so we prepared a large lunch of smoked salmon and roast chicken – only to learn that she is a vegetarian. (As I discovered later, rather to my sorrow, this is often the preference of midwives.) Aware that some vegetarians don't balk at eating fish, I asked, 'How about a bit of smoked salmon?' 'Nothing that wiggles,' said Mrs Kitzinger firmly. That resolved, Sally set about reconstituting the lunch while we talked.

Sheila (as I was soon calling her) was well worth the effort. She had just returned from a visit to Russia, where she was downright appalled at the treatment of women in the maternity wards – and this in a country where more than 90 per cent of doctors are women. Far from being angels of mercy – or even kind, solicitous supporters of the women in their care – these female obstetricians were as rigid and insensitive as many of their much-criticised male counterparts in Western countries. They energetically enforced a system, long discredited in all other industrialised countries, of total exclusion of fathers from the maternity ward for the week to ten days during which the mother was confined. Crowded together in the ward, the mothers would wait until the doctors had left and then dash to the windows and throw down notes to their husbands waiting below: 'Ivan, we have a baby girl!' or 'Please send up some fruit,' and so on. If a nurse came in and caught them doing it, she would slam the window shut; but as soon as she left, they were at it again. 'They're like naughty girls in a school dorm,' said Sheila.

(But it does cause one to reflect on the generally accepted view that male domination is responsible for the many indignities visited upon women in childbirth. Could there also be another component – that regardless of gender, absolute power wielded over the powerless in enclosed institutions such as prisons, insane asylums, and hospitals creates the potential for abuse?)

In England, Sheila Kitzinger's unflagging championship of natural childbirth has produced some spectacular results, chiefly in the humanisation of most British hospitals. Since her first book, *The Experience of Childbirth*, was published in 1962, many disagreeable routine procedures have vanished for ever – for example, the ordeal of 'prepping', meaning the shaving of the mother's pubic hair, administering an enema, and strapping her legs into stirrups. Fathers, once banished from the delivery room, are now encouraged to turn up for the event, and they do so in droves. One of Sheila's most successful achievements has been the drastic reduction of episiotomies. In her view, forcefully advanced in her books on the subject, this painful and sometimes dangerous cut is usually quite unnecessary, its usefulness limited to the very occasional emergency such as a difficult breech birth or foetal distress.

In spite of all these undeniable achievements, there has been a distinct backlash in England against the Kitzinger-inspired natural birth movement, described in a series of articles by Polly Toynbee in the *Guardian*. While Ms Toynbee gave full marks to Sheila Kitzinger for all she has done ('Her *Good Birth Guide* has obstetricians up and down the land quaking. If Britain is now one of the most progressive countries in obstetrical practice, it is largely due to her'), she gave equal space to the counter-viewpoint. In an article with the cruel – but telling – headline 'Natural Childbirth, a Child of the Sixties, Was and is Largely a Nutty Fad from a Noisy Group of Lentil-Eating Earth Goddesses,' she went full tilt in favour of the anti-natural-childbirth lobby, organised by Maureen Treadwell, a teacher and elected official on her local council.

There is something to be said for the Toynbee/Treadwell position, the main point of which is that many women have been conned into believing that if they follow the precepts of natural childbirth, the event can be (in Sheila Kitzinger's words) 'a life-enhancing personal experience in which they can get in touch with their own feelings and give glad expression to the energy sweeping through their bodies'. Polly Toynbee, speaking from experience as a mother of three, wrote that 'squatting and yelling and delivering in baths may suit some, but others are very grateful for a good old hospital bed, a reassuring doctor and a needle-full of something nice to take the pain away'. Maureen Treadwell has had hundreds of letters from women full of stories of their horrible treatment in the name of 'natural childbirth', many saying how guilty they feel for having failed to give birth naturally.

I asked Sheila about this development. 'I've debated with her on television, but it was frustrating – never enough time to discuss these matters thoroughly.'

Actually, Sheila Kitzinger is by no means as doctrinaire as Polly Toynbee's articles might imply. For example, in *The Complete Book of Pregnancy and Childbirth* (1985), a large illustrated tome full of basic information and practical advice, she has described various anaesthetics used in hospitals and gives a non-judgmental, unbiased account of epidurals – Polly Toynbee's 'needle-full of something nice to take the pain away'. Sheila has noted that 'an epidural can provide complete relief from pain and can even be used as an anaesthetic for a Caesarean section ... For a painful labour which is difficult or prolonged, it seems the perfect answer. Many women have said how marvellous the epidural was, but it should be your own choice.' Throughout the book, her theme is informed freedom of choice – which should, after all, be the ultimate goal.

While I have great admiration for Sheila Kitzinger and her like-minded cohorts in the United States, I should admit that some of their rhetoric seems more than a trifle highfalutin' and overblown. Sheila Kitzinger, on the role of the midwife:

Midwives have always been mediators between nature and culture. They deal with blood and body fluids, and with human beings at our first raw, elemental moment of existence. They have to be able to understand feelings which are passionate and basic.

Lucky for the rest of us that some actually rather like dealing in blood and body fluids – which would certainly not be my cup of tea.

One theme that reverberates throughout the literature of midwives is *bonding*, a subject that fills me with uneasiness.

We are told over and over in midwifery texts, journals, and books that the expectant mother should first bond with the midwife – and so should the baby's father (although nothing is said about the danger of *that* bond going too far) – and, above all, bond with the newborn baby. The infant, as soon as delivered, should be put right on the mother's breast for instant bonding.

To me, that all sounds like a bit of claptrap. Common sense would advise establishing a friendly and companionable relationship with the midwife, as with anyone else with whom one is working towards a common goal. As to the newborn: if it is, in fact, whisked off to be washed and tidied up, or taken to some remote incubator in the hospital nursery, will this endanger the whole future relationship of mother and child?

The bonding advocates have overlooked the fact that new mothers, like the rest of the population, are individuals with distinct preferences and dislikes. Thus while Ms A. may get pleasure from the newborn, all fresh, slimy, and blood-streaked put to suckle, while its father cuts the umbilical cord, Ms B. might prefer to wait until her baby has at least been given a bath, wrapped up, and put in a nappy – and her squeamish husband might turn pale at the suggestion that he be the cord-cutter. And what about adopted children whom the new parents may never have set eyes on until they are several months – or even years – old? Are they to be cast into some unbonded limbo in which they are destined to languish for ever without benefit of true, deep parental affection?

Whatever is meant by 'bonding' (epoxy comes to mind), it seems obvious that those first allegedly precious moments have very little to do with the eventual relationship of mother and child. The mother may well come unglued when the baby is a naughty two-year-old or a difficult teenager. She and her child may or may not eventually become great friends; if 'bonding' is instant, true compatibility may take a lifetime, as in the development of any lasting friendship.

That said – and I did have to get it off my chest at some point – my tour of the American midwifery scene was most illuminating, from the remembrances of Southern grannies to the experiences of latter-day practitioners.

Chapter 10

GRANNIES

Throughout the Deep South, countless generations of poor rural women, both white and black, were attended in childbirth by 'granny midwives', mostly black women whose skills were handed down from mother to daughter over the centuries. Now banished from the scene, outlawed in the mid-1970s when medical boards in the Southern states prohibited their practice, the grannies have faded into the collective memory of recent history.

Asking around in 1990 about this vanished species (Were they an asset to their communities? Should they be legally reinstated today, when obstetrical services are almost non-existent in the rural South?), I got a wide range of answers. George Purdue, a black representative in the Alabama legislature, had consulted his mother just before our meeting: 'I had breakfast with her, that's why I was a little bit late. And she told me that I was four pounds ten ounces, a low-birth-weight baby. I was delivered by a granny midwife, at home in 1943.' His mother was ever grateful to the midwife, who had brought life-saving skills to the birth scene. A knowledgeable advocate of maternal and child welfare in all its ramifications, Mr Purdue thinks there may well be a need for the return of trained lay midwives in the vastly underserved rural South.

By contrast, white health workers in Montgomery with whom I spoke were unanimously opposed to the grannies. The physicians saw them as a bane and a scourge, largely responsible for the high maternal/infant death rate in Alabama – which seems odd, considering that the death rate some fifteen years after the abolition of the grannies remains one of the highest in the nation. A public-health nurse – too young to have had any contact with the grannies – wrinkled her nose in disgust: 'They were filthy, ignorant old women.' But, I asked, didn't they have to pass fairly extensive tests in the 1930s and 1940s to qualify for a licence? 'The only test I know of was the Wasserman test, ha-ha, tee-hee,' she giggled, the Wasserman being a test for syphilis.

Seeking to sort fact from fiction, I found in *Motherwit: An Alabama Midwife's Story* (New York: Dutton, 1989) by Onnie Lee Logan as told to Katherine Clark, a useful guide to the actual life and times of the granny midwife. Mrs Logan, born in 1910, worked as a midwife for many years, first as a young girl assisting her mother and later on her own. In 1947, when she applied for a state licence to practise in Mobile County, she had to go through a nine-month training programme and then submit to rigorous supervision from the board of health for annual renewal of her permit.

Mrs Logan may have put her finger on one important reason for the medical profession's campaign against the grannies. As long as she was attending poor black women, she said, the doctors didn't care. But after she started delivering white girls – 'nice, outstanding white girls, then that's when they started complaining. Said I was taking their money. In fact that's what they said. My patients have come and told me what the doctors said.'

An interesting sidelight on the rise and fall of granny midwives was furnished by Mrs Mary Lee Parker, a white woman born in the early years of the century. I visited her in Montgomery with Dawn Cox, a young public-health worker of that city.

Long widowed, Mrs Parker is now totally crippled by degenerative arthritis. She met us in a wheelchair on the ground floor of her large house, where she lives alone; she can no longer manage the stairs to the upper storeys. As she described her early training as a public-health nurse, and later her work with the granny midwives of Alabama, one glimpsed the bright, adventurous girl from Georgia, determined to make her mark in her chosen field.

'I didn't like hospital work and I didn't like private duty,' she said. 'I realised that what I really wanted was some background in public-health nursing.'

In the 1920s and 1930s there were no training facilities for this occupation in the South, so she applied to Columbia University, was accepted, and went to live in New York – in itself a daring move for a Southern teenager. At first, there were some awkward moments. 'The teacher called on me to tell something about the food we had in rural Georgia. I was so scared; I had never been out of Georgia before. So my knees started hitting and I got up and I said, "The chief diet of these people were fat, doughy biscuits and gravy, with plenty of syrup." And when I said "syrup" everybody's jaw fell. So I said, "I know up here you all say 'see-rup', but where I come from we say 'surrup'." And that kind of broke the ice.'

After a year at Columbia, Mrs Parker joined the teaching staff at the New York Maternity Center, where she held regular prenatal sessions for pregnant women, instructing them in nutrition, baby care, and the like. She also assisted doctors at deliveries. The clientele was varied, some well-to-do, others very poor. 'I had a black lady whose husband was vice-president of the New York Life Insurance Company . . . a lot of women whose husbands worked in the ship-yards . . . foreign girls, immigrants who couldn't speak English.' She remembered a young Turkish woman whose tradition called for swaddling the baby's legs very tightly so they wouldn't grow crooked. The baby was screaming: 'I talked to the mother in sign language, trying to explain with my hands. I took off the wrapping, and the baby stopped crying. The mother immediately got the idea. You had to do things that way in those days.'

Tired of New York (and possibly homesick for doughy biscuits and sur-rup), Mrs Parker wrote to the State of Alabama, explaining that she was looking for a position in public-health nursing, specifi-cally in prenatal care and childbirth. She moved to Montgomery in 1931, after a three-month internship in Opelika, where she learned the Alabama health department's rules, regulations, and procedures.

Her assignment: to provide prenatal care in rural clinics run by the health department, and to supervise the education of granny midwives to enable them to pass a public-health exam, needed for state licensure.

'At that time we had seventeen hundred granny midwives in the state,' she said. 'Another nurse had been teaching them, but she was getting ready to retire. I was twenty-seven years old, and I'd had some experience with granny midwife work years before in Georgia so they asked me to take over.' One of the first things she did was to arrange for women prisoners serving time in local jails to make hospital-style caps and gowns for the grannies, whom she also provided with medical kits containing all the necessaries of their occupation, such as scissors, basins, soap, towels, eye drops for the newborn, and a baby scale.

Aside from providing her students with these much appreciated – and highly practical – accoutrements of their calling, Parker introduced other innovations: 'I acquired a movie projector and films on pregnancy and normal delivery, which I showed to the midwives.' Eventually, she had an incubator in every county health department, as well as a portable incubator to transport premature infants to a hospital.

Although her home was now in Montgomery, she spent a huge amount of time on the road, travelling in a van containing the movie gear, educational material dealing with all aspects of pregnancy and birth, and medical supplies. 'I went to every county in the state. We had meetings in all of them, and I would have all the midwives come in. Most of the midwives were black, except up in the northern part of the state, where they were mixed. We had very few white ones in the southern counties.'

Requirements for licensure were fairly stiff, including a written exam, monthly inspection of the midwife's equipment bag and her home, and attendance at monthly meetings run by the local public-health nurse. Many of the older midwives were illiterate: 'I asked them if they wouldn't like to give up the work, because although they may have been good at their job, they hadn't a prayer of fulfilling the requirements for a licence. They agreed to drop out of the programme, although some no doubt continued to help neighbour women as they had always done.'

After she had weeded out 'the illiterate and those not receptive to learning' from the seventeen hundred grannies who had been practising in Alabama when she came on the scene, there remained five hundred granny or lay midwives who were well trained, well equipped, and knowledgeable. Some of Mrs Parker's students were highly educated; one had a master's degree; many had been teachers

and other professionals before going into midwifery. Yet the stereotype of 'ignorant, filthy old women' persisted. A *Life* magazine article
of December 3, 1951, describing in *Life*'s inimitable style the successful delivery of a baby by a certified nurse-midwife, observed, 'The
new midwife had succeeded in a situation where the fast-disappearing
"granny" midwife of the South, armed with superstition and a pair
of rusty scissors, might have killed both mother and child.'

The really spectacular feature of Mrs Parker's work in Alabama
arose from her connection with Tuskegee Institute, founded by
Booker T. Washington as an all-black enclave of higher learning in
the segregated South. Tuskegee specialised in research and education
in agriculture, home economics, mechanical engineering – and nurse
training, with its own hospital, doctors, paediatricians, and nurse-
midwives.

'Every year I took twenty-five women there, my best midwives
chosen from different counties around the state. Every summer I
would take a different group. We stayed in the dormitory: they got
to see both hospital deliveries and home deliveries out in the
country.' After their stint at Tuskegee, the midwives would return
home to spread the knowledge they had acquired among their fellow
practitioners.

If one thinks back to the deplorable history of the Deep South in
the 1930s, unrelieved generalised racism punctuated by lynchings
and other horrors visited by the white population against blacks, the
sheer boldness of a young white Southern girl taking this route is
fairly astonishing – as was her acceptance by the all-black Tuskegee
personnel. Somehow, Mrs Parker seems to have been born mercifully
colour blind; in our conversation, her affection and appreciation for
the black women with whom she worked came through loud and
strong. A natural storyteller like so many Southerners, she described
many a 'beautiful delivery' by a granny whom she was observing.
'The nurse-midwife at Tuskegee,' she said, 'was a glorious person.
She passed away last year, but she was listed in Alabama as one of
the most promising women.' 'Was she a black woman?' 'Yes, she
was. Gotha Wilkerson was a wonderful person.'

Chapter 11

CERTIFIED NURSE-MIDWIVES

In America, midwives fall into two distinct categories. There are certified nurse-midwives, who after decades of uphill striving are now recognised and licensed in all fifty states. They are registered nurses with additional training in midwifery. They function as adjuncts to obstetrical personnel in hospitals, subordinate to the physicians in charge. Today, CNMs are much sought after in many (but by no means all) obstetrical facilities. In general they do not officiate at home births – which are frowned on by their medical superiors – although some rebellious free spirits in the ranks continue to do so, often at some risk to their professional status.

In contrast, the direct-entry midwife's underlying philosophy is that in more than 90 per cent of cases childbirth is a natural procedure in which medical intervention is not only unnecessary, but often harmful. Her interest, and practice, is in attending family-centred home births for those women who prefer this route. Her clients are for the most part well-educated women, versed in feminist literature and determined to avoid the male-dominated world of the hospital.

In Europe, there is no such creature as a 'nurse-midwife.' As Dr Marsden Wagner of the World Health Organization put it, midwifery and nursing are two entirely separate (and highly regarded) professions, each trained in specific skills. The requirement that a midwife must first get a degree in nursing would be akin, he said, to demanding that a plumber in order to be licensed should first pass the necessary tests to qualify as a carpenter.

From Lani Rosenberger, a midwife who had years of experience delivering babies in home births, I learned something of the training needed to become a çertified nurse-midwife. She had reluctantly decided to go that route because of the ever-present danger of harassment in states where direct-entry midwifery is outlawed as 'practising medicine without a licence'.

In terms of the length of time required to become a certified nurse-midwife, she said, 'They tell you that it only takes a few years to be certified, but in reality, it takes two to four years to become a registered nurse; then, to get into a CNM school, you must have a BA or BS (some require an MA or MS); then you must have two years' experience in labour and delivery. But no one will give you a job in L and D until you've had two years' experience in Medical/Surgical, so that's four more years, then CNM school is eighteen months to two years. That's a minimum of ten years – in ten years, I could be an OB!'

What about the nursing school curriculum? 'Nursing school does teach certain basic skills – for example, taking a pulse and blood pressure; collecting and preparing specimens for lab tests; auscultating heart and lungs – which are rudimentary procedures for all nurses, doctors, midwives, dentists, veterinarians in their respective spheres of practice. But of those professionals, only midwives are required to take nursing courses before studying their chosen profession. The few skills taught in nursing schools that apply to midwifery could easily be learned in a weekend workshop.'

But there must be *something* useful to be gained from those years in nursing school, I insisted. Precious little, it seems. Pressed for examples, she came up with some categories:

Useful
  Basic physiology
  Microbiology – study of microbes
  Physical assessment – examination of a patient (or client, in
    midwife's terms) for general health
  General pharmacology – only marginally useful, as midwives
    don't as a rule administer drugs

Not Useful – irrelevant to midwifery
Gerontology – physiological and pathological phenomena
associated with old age
Physiology of disease
Cutting up a dead cat and a human cadaver; putting together
a human skeleton
Surgical nursing
Psychiatric nursing
Nursing theory

All the 'useful' items listed above are already included in the
extensive special training required in states where direct-entry
midwives are licensed. Furthermore, they are part of the curriculum
of midwife associations in states such as California and New York,
where direct-entry midwives have established their own rigorous
standards for self-accreditation, as part of their effort to achieve
legal status.

The chequered history of the certified nurse-midwives' upward climb
to professional status is set forth in *Nurse-Midwifery in America*, the
1986 report of the Nurse-Midwives Foundation.

From it we learn that the first US nurse-midwifery training programme was started by the Maternity Center Association in New
York City, in 1931, where Mrs Mary Parker got her start. In the
1930s and 1940s, four more programmes were established, but it was
not until 1955 that the American College of Nurse-Midwives was
incorporated, its objective 'to evaluate and approve Certified Nurse-
Midwife services and education programmes'. By 1982, certified
nurse-midwives were conducting deliveries in every state except
Idaho, Indiana, and North Dakota. Today, certified nurse-midwives
are licensed to practise in all fifty states.

In preparing *Nurse-Midwifery in America*, the editors sent out a
nationwide questionnaire to all practising certified nurse-midwives.
Under the section 'Hindrance to the Practice of Midwifery', the
report summarised, as a principal hindrance, 'too many physicians
concerned about loss of income from Certified Nurse-Midwife practitioners', followed by 'lack of acceptance from community MDs of

nurse-midwifery as a worthwhile profession'. Some of the individual replies to the questionnaire underlined these 'hindrances':

The OB/GYNs see the CNMs as a financial threat. Our medical back-up is only for an identified population – indigent and low risk. (CNM, Florida)

Many MDs are quite outspoken about how they think I've hit their pocket. (CNM, Montana)

This is the underlying reason for most of our problems. We are a middle-class private practice in direct competition for paying patients with MDs. (CNM, California)

As to the second hindrance – lack of acceptance of nurse-midwifery by MDs – the respondents had these comments:

There is open hostility by most OB/GYNs in the community overtly expressing that they do not want to see CNMs practicing in the area. (CNM, Ohio)

My practice is more 'tolerated' than accepted. (CNM, California)

MDs generally are unaware of or unaccepting of CNMs as professionals. Many resent the fact that we know normal obstetrics as well or sometimes better than they do. (CNM, Texas)

The Federal Trade Commission weighed in heavily on the side of the midwives – rather to my surprise, as its performance as a consumer watchdog agency has too often been sadly lacklustre and ineffective, with a tendency to lean over backwards to avoid offending major business interests.

Commissioner Patricia Bailey explained the FTC's position:

The underlying premise for all of the Commission's health-care activities is our conviction that competition in the delivery of health care is profoundly in the public interest: it will foster innovative approaches to the delivery of health care and provide consumers with a choice of treatment alternatives – probably at lowered cost and without any adverse effect on the quality of care provided.

Right there, Commissioner Bailey summarised several very touchy issues for the profit-hungry medical industry: competition in the public interest, innovative approaches, consumer choice of treatment alternatives, lower costs. Fighting words, backed up by FTC initiatives.

Eventually the certified nurse-midwives won the blessing – sort of – of the super-prestigious American College of Obstetricians and Gynecologists. In a joint statement by ACOG and the American College of Nurse-Midwives (1982), principles of the relationship of the two groups were set forth. This brief document made clear who would rule the roost: 'The maternity care team should be directed by a qualified obstetrician/gynecologist ... Quality of care is enhanced by the interdependent practice of the obstetrician/gynecologist and certified nurse-midwife working in a relationship of mutual respect, trust and professional responsibility. *This does not necessarily imply the physical presence of the physician when care is being given by the certified nurse-midwife.*' (Emphasis added.)

In a nutshell, the certified nurse-midwife must follow directions of the obstetrician, but if the fellow doesn't happen to show up for the birth, she is in charge. How does this work in practice?

At the national headquarters of the American College of Nurse-Midwives in Washington, DC, on April 10, 1990, I met with three board members of that organisation: Karen Fennell, government relations director; Jan Kriebs, board member; and Mary Ellen Bouchard, a practising CNM.

Like all good organisational advocates, they plied me with reams of printed material – policy statements, newsletters, law review articles. In our discussion, I was mainly interested in exploring three areas:

The impact of Federal Trade Commission intervention on behalf of CNMs – how effective has it been?

The college's policy regarding direct-entry midwives.

How the physician/CNM collaboration works out in practice.

The FTC's support of the midwives has done much to alert the certified nurse-midwives to their rights when faced with physician opposition, said Karen Fennell. 'Our members call me and ask, "Where can I find a good lawyer who knows about FTC regulations?

I believe there's been restraint of trade in my practice," and they go out and hire lawyers.'

From discussions with direct-entry midwives around the country, I had got the impression that they and the certified nurse-midwives were very much at odds with each other. CNMs, I was told, are implacably opposed to the whole concept of lay midwifery and home birth – the idea of untutored, untrained women muscling in on the territory of those who, having gone through years of expensive professional training, have won the right to be licensed.

While this mutual hostility may well exist in some areas, I found no evidence of it at the national level. The American College of Nurse-Midwives has never denounced lay midwifery or home birth; on the contrary, the college's only 'position statement' on the subject (August 1989) states, 'The ACNM will actively explore, through the Division of Accreditation, the testing on non-nurse professional midwifery educational routes.' Jan Kriebs told me she knows that direct-entry midwifery works and that she is personally all for it. She has sat in on board examinations in states where direct-entry midwives are granted licences and found the requirements to be exemplary, the exams 'quite rigorous'.

As to CNM/obstetrician relationships, Mary Ellen Bouchard was particularly forthcoming on the subject of 'difficult births'. While this phrase usually refers to an adverse physical condition of mother and/or unborn child, the difficulties described by Ms Bouchard were entirely between CNMs and physicians.

Her first 'difficult birth' took place shortly after she got out of midwifery school and got a job in central Massachusetts. 'Everything was fine and hunky-dory until we started having our first private payers come in. And all hell broke loose including fights in the middle of delivery – a screaming fight in the middle of the hospital hallway. Finally, that's where I discovered at two in the morning what the real issue was, when the doctor just came in and took over my patient – economics. He said, "You have private payers and you're not supposed to have those." Apparently the physicians assumed we'd only take Medicaid patients.'

In another incident, 'the physician came in and tried to take over the birth. He handled the woman very roughly – and her husband almost decked him.' At issue was whether or not the woman should have an episiotomy, with the objective of speeding up labour for the doctor's convenience. An unequal confrontation developed, the wife and her husband refusing the episiotomy, backed up by the delivery nurse and CNM Bouchard. 'The physician was a tad enraged and I literally had to throw myself across the bed to separate the patient from the physician. So he stormed out and left. The baby was wonderful, they had a great birth. But as a result of that situation, the whole thing came to a head. Within two weeks, I was dismissed, and the midwifery service closed within a year's time.'

Mary Welcome, a certified nurse-midwife employed by Southtown County General Hospital in Georgia*, told me about her training, why she chose this line of work, changes she has seen in the practice, and some of the difficulties she has encountered.

The initial impetus was supplied by the birth of her own son, Sam, in 1973, on the whole a bleak and unpleasant experience. 'I really didn't like the way I was treated,' she said. 'I never saw the same doctor twice, they were never very friendly – they never answered any of my questions. Everything I learned about the birth process was through reading.' During her labour, the nurses were equally unhelpful; they barely entered the room, and tried to kick her husband out. 'He insisted on staying. I had decided on unanaesthetised birth, but back in those days the nurses couldn't understand anyone wanting to be awake for delivery.' Then and there, she determined to become a midwife.

First she went to nursing school, and from 1975 to 1978 worked as a labour and delivery nurse in another hospital. In this capacity she observed changes in medically mandated procedures and techniques. By the time she came on the scene, the rage for forceps delivery – routinely used for the great majority of births in the 1950s – had subsided.

Mary Welcome went to the University of Mississippi Medical School for her nurse-midwifery training, where she worked in hospitals and clinics – no home births because 'none of the physicians wanted to take the liability of doing that'. There were a couple of

* Her name and that of the hospital where she works have been changed at her request.

CNMs in Jackson doing home births, she said, but this practice stopped when their back-up physician had to quit because of pressure from the obstetrical community.

As Mary sees it, the essential role of a certified nurse-midwife is that of 'patient advocate'. While CNMs are basically under the jurisdiction of the hospital, bound by conditions of their employment to obey rules set down by their physician bosses, there is in fact plenty of leeway for the CNM to use her own discretion – particularly since the obstetricians, having employed the CNMs for the long haul of overseeing many boring hours of labour, tend to be but fleeting presences on the scene.

Mary added, 'I will help the women I see to get up and walk. I try to do as little intervention as possible, try to keep the IVs out, keep the medication away, give them their babies to nurse, and try to do the kind of things the doctors aren't even there for. You know, they come and deliver the baby and then they are – tchoo! gone.'

The certified nurse-midwife who has followed the patient through-out the lengthy prenatal care sessions, in which they discuss all aspects of pregnancy through birth and on to the first days of mother-hood, may proffer a 'Birth Plan' to the mother-to-be on which she can state what she does/doesn't want to happen at the end of the road. 'A typical birth plan might say she wants no IVs, no electronic foetal monitoring, would like to get up and walk around freely, be able to drink liquids, would prefer not to have an episiotomy, would like the baby with her as much as possible. Just simple things like that.'

Somehow, the birth plan of one of Mary's patients fell into the hands of the hospital business manager, who told Mary that 'we are not going to abide by this. We are going to kick her out.' Mary pointed out that the woman was due in two weeks: 'You can't kick her out.'

Why did he care – and what concern was it of his? I asked.

'Well, he felt that it would be bad for business to have this demanding type of person in their practice.' Mary warned the woman that she might get a phone call from the business manager, and that she should ignore it. 'And I had to plead with the doctors and say, listen, we'll handle this woman, she'll do fine.' As it turned out, the patient delivered her baby twenty minutes after arrival, with no IV and no monitor. All the in-fighting with the business manager was just another annoying pinprick in the life of a certified nurse-midwife.

Mary led me through the labyrinth of charges and pay scales – how they are allocated among the professional staff, CNMs and obstetricians; who cares for which patients; the striking double standard of treatment meted out to the paying patients and the indigents.

Unlike most county hospitals, which cater almost exclusively to the very poor, Southtown County General has a large number of paying patients who come in through the offices of private physicians. At the time of our interview, there were ten obstetricians in private practice and about fifty indigent women delivering each month. Formerly, the ten doctors would parcel these out so that each had five non-paying patients. 'Needless to say,' Mary continued, 'the doctors resisted – resented the heck out of this. They felt it was unfair, they were practising medicine for nothing. And, you know, when you charge what they charge, to do anything for free is abhorrent. So they essentially threatened to leave Southtown County General unless something was done to correct this problem of the non-paying people.'

The corrective measure, it seems, was the hiring of certified nurse-midwives to look after the indigents.

For this service, the hospital pays the CNM an annual wage of $42,000 – augmented by her work for the private patients, for which the doctor pays her an additional $600 per case. 'We CNMs have a very small percentage of those, average four to five a month.' Mary's annual salary – hospital wage plus private patients – comes to about $52,000, from which she pays $5,000 malpractice insurance.

The doctor's fee for a normal, uncomplicated birth is $2,200, to which the paying patient must add another $2,000 or $3,000 for her hospital bill. At that, for her $600, the CNM does all the care and delivery: 'We may or may not ever call the doctor, and he may or may not ever see our private patients.' The doctor's justification for the gap between the $600 for the CNM and the $2,200 billed to the patient is that 50 per cent of his bill goes to pay the overhead of his office, used by CNMs for prenatal care of the paying patients.

However, the doctor's fee for the paying patient also includes $400 for lab work, such as ultrasound technology. So the final reckoning is something like this:

Fee to doctor	$2,200
Lab work	−400
Doctor now has	$1,800
and pays the CNM	$600

The doctor ends up with $1,200, although he may never actually attend his patient's accouchement*.

As 'patient advocates', the certified nurse-midwives find that their non-intervention policy works well. Their Caesarean rate is about 14 per cent, as compared with 25 per cent for the hospital as a whole. 'All breech babies are automatically considered candidates for C-section,' Mary said – but once in a while one will slip through and escape the knife: 'Becky, one of our CNMs, called the doctor and said, "We have this breech baby, and it's just about here." The doctor came rushing in, called the operating room crew, and just before they arrived the girl delivered her baby, which was just fine. That's the only way you can sneak a breech by without the mother having an unnecessary operation.'

The unkindest cut of all is the episiotomy – cutting through the vulva. 'Many of our doctors believe you have to use Pitocin on everyone, everyone needs an epidural, and you have to cut a huge episiotomy right through the rectum and pull the baby out,' Mary Welcome said. 'It's called an episioproctotonomy.'

CNMs, coming from a different perspective on the whole labour scene, seldom perform this supremely unpleasant operation. Mary says she delivers 90 per cent of the babies without cutting: 'I'll occasionally cut if there is foetal distress. If the baby is sitting there in the birth canal and the heart tones are down, the woman is pushing and it's not coming, I'll cut just to speed it up.'

The clinic patients, whose racial composition reflects that of the county as a whole – unlike that of inner-city general hospitals, about

* These figures, for 1989, have doubtless increased over the last several years.

two-thirds white – range all the way from those entitled to Medicaid to women who drop in off the streets already in labour. Most doctors refuse to accept any Medicaid patients; some might see one or two a month.

The indigents get 'the absolute bare minimum', Mary said. 'They are discriminated against in every way. They get the ward room, for one thing, a three-bed room that has no shower in it. Because they are never given a private room, they can't have rooming-in with their baby. They can't have an epidural even if they want one.'

Many of the clinic patients are high-school dropouts, un-demanding types, non-complainers with no concept of what their rights are vis-à-vis the hospital set-up. As 'patient advocate', Mary is often at odds with the authorities: 'When they get to Southtown County General they're not given the same privileges as the other people. In fact, doctors have even said things like, "That's a clinic patient in the private delivery room. I want you to put her in the recovery room, because I have a private one coming in, and my patient is paying and yours isn't."'

At one point, there was a move afoot to establish separate waiting rooms for the families of indigent and paying patients: 'The adminis-tration came up to me and they said, "Mary, how would you feel if we had a separate area for y'all's patients?" I said, "A separate area?" And they said, "Well, you know, a separate fathers' waiting room for the clinic people and another for the private paying people, because it's really getting out of hand in that waiting room" – mean-ing that very often when indigent patients come in they have a lot of relatives who take up space. I just said, "I feel that's discriminating, isn't that like the separate toilets for white and black?"'

Finally I edged into the possibly thorny question of lay/direct-entry midwives and home births. After all, the certified nurse-midwives have spent many years and dollars to achieve professional status. Do they feel any hostility toward the lay midwife, who plies her trade without benefit of academic schooling?

'There are some among the very staunchest of the nurse-midwives who feel that way, and I'm not one of them,' said Mary. 'I think it's great that we have lay midwives, and that if a woman wants to have a home birth there's someone she can call.' What about apprenticeship in lieu of a structured college of midwifery? 'You mean lay midwives who do apprentice work? I think it's excellent,' Mary said. 'I think that after you've done a hundred deliveries, if you have a little bit of theory along with it, that would be sufficient. The main thing about birth is the experience of knowing what to do in difficult situations and anticipating what might go wrong. Experience is the whole thing.'

Chapter 12

THE FARM

Wishing to discover the fountainhead of modern direct-entry midwifery, I spent two days in April 1989 at the Farm in Tennessee visiting Ina May Gaskin, acknowledged foremost theoretician and practitioner of the movement in America.

To prepare for our discussion, with a heavy heart I dipped into her 1977 book *Spiritual Midwifery* – its off-putting title followed by a text written in the vernacular of Haight-Ashbury flower children. The first 220 pages is all ecstatic moms telling it like it is, rhapsodising over the blissful experience of labour *à la* Gaskin: 'I realised that if I loosened up the pain would go away and everything would be psychedelic and Holy.' 'I was somewhere on the astral plane, feeling all the forces of the Universe, it felt like, pounding my body. It was like my body was its own thing.' 'Having a baby was the heaviest thing that ever happened to me. I felt God creating life through me, and I felt that I was God.'

This is followed, however, by 200 pages of essential advice for the aspirant midwife – step by step through prenatal sessions, the birth, the care of the mother and newborn. At that, one is sometimes brought up short, as in this passage, where Gaskin wrote, 'I spread open her puss with my fingers,' to which she appended a footnote: '"Vagina" is the medical term, a Latin word, but I prefer to use "puss" because it sounds friendlier. You may mentally substitute whatever word you like.'

The Farm owes its origins to the utopian vision of Stephen Gaskin, Ina May's husband. In the 1960s Gaskin, an instructor at San Francisco State College, became a magnet for upwards of a thousand

devoted young disciples, who flocked to his regular Monday-night
class for instruction in Zen, mysticism, and related spiritual subjects,
followed by after-school treats such as all-night pot parties, then the
height of fashion for the Haight-Ashbury hippie crowd.

By 1970, Gaskin had decided that the urban academic life was no
longer for him. While on a nationwide lecture tour he had spotted
a 1,700-acre tract of cheap fertile land in northern Tennessee. On
Columbus Day, 1970, he set out with Ina May, then aged thirty, and
hundreds of the hippie faithful, who had assembled all manner of
vehicles – old school buses, vans, campers, trailers – on a circuitous
odyssey of 6,000 miles, stopping at various universities, parks, and
churches along the way. Seven months later, in May 1971, the Gaskins and assorted flower children arrived in the tiny hamlet of Summertown to take possession of their new abode.

During the next decade thousands of seekers after spiritual guidance flocked to the Summertown commune, some for brief visits
and others to stay on as permanent members. By 1979 the Farm's
population had swollen from its original 250 to 1,500. At first, money
wasn't much of a problem, as members of the collective agreed to
pool all their worldly goods. The real difficulty arose from their
collective ignorance of the rudiments of farming, so that the dream
of living off the bounty of Mother Earth soon faded. The one successful crop was soybeans; those who wearied of an unrelieved diet
of this wholesome but undeniably dull fare began to drift away, until
by the mid-1980s the collective (its organisational structure changed
in 1983 to a cooperative) had shrunk back to about 250 hardy, hungry
souls.

Three of us made the trek to the Farm: Betty Corbett, a charming
young Southern woman pregnant with her first baby; Ted Kalman,
who knows all the proper medical terms and is thoroughly familiar
with the midwife philosophy; and I, neophyte, anxious to learn all I
could about the, to me, obscure routines of midwifery.

Access to the Farm is not easy. A plane to Nashville, a rented
car, 65 miles of winding country roads with confusing signposts,
finally a small reception building with a sign instructing visitors
to stop for identification before proceeding to the Farm. We
stopped; nobody was at home, so we proceeded along a bumpy,

unpaved road flanked by fields full of weeds until we reached the Gaskins' dwelling.

Their spacious living-room-cum-kitchen is full of the paraphernalia of the cooperative's transformation from a utopian dream to the entrepreneurial real world. These erstwhile tillers of the soil have long since abandoned the farming venture (except for the soybean products, which we had ample opportunity to sample at each meal) and are now into, as they would put it, electronics, computers, word processing, desktop publishing, portable radiation detectors, and other profitable enterprises. Stephen Gaskin, his long hair and beard now snow-white – the only remnants of his former hippie persona – presides over some of the mercantile aspects of current Farm life. Indoctrination into Eastern mysticism has faded away, and LSD is passé. These days, I was told, any use of drugs or alcohol is frowned on by the Farm cooperative.

As for Ina May, if you can't judge a book by its cover, you certainly can't judge this writer by her published work. In real life, she is mercifully devoid of the sort of mushy malarky that I found so disheartening in *Spiritual Midwifery*. From her no-nonsense appearance – plain and neat, with upright posture, she could have stepped out of a Grant Wood portrait – to her extremely cogent and informative conversation, she was all one could have hoped for as a guide to the complexities of latter-day midwifery.

Ina May's entrée into what was to become her life's career occurred on the journey from California to Tennessee, during which three babies were born to members of the group.

'The first birth took place in the parking lot of Northwestern University, Illinois. All I did was watch – I didn't handle the baby. The mother, who was plain, became strikingly beautiful – I couldn't take my eyes off her. I was thrilled.' The second birth happened a few days later, in a tiny, crowded bus. This time, Ina May decided to act as midwife. She was reading a midwifery manual when a woman snatched it away: 'She was superstitious, and she thought that if I read the part about what you do if the baby doesn't breathe, I would make it happen.' In the event, the baby was born dark blue and didn't breathe until given the kiss of life (CPR) by Stephen, who came dashing over. The baby survived and is today an honours student;

but the terror of that experience was enough to send Ina May racing back to the manual.

By the time of the third birth, Ina May had virtually memorised the book. The next baby was born in the tiny hamlet of Ripley, New York, where at the onset of labour the expectant parents had pulled over and parked on the side of the main street. State troopers came alongside: 'They were so eager not to have to do this birth themselves that they begged us to tell them what we needed. And I said, "Yes, we need some cord clamp (for the umbilical cord) and a place to park," all of which they quickly arranged.' As Ina May was well aware that lay midwifery is illegal in New York State, the cooperation of these stalwart law enforcers was most reassuring. There was yet another good omen: it was near Christmas, and across the street townspeople were practising Christmas carols. When they heard the baby had been born, they rang all the church bells as a welcome.

The caravan, its population now augmented by the three new-borns, set out for Rhode Island. By the time it arrived the story of the Christmas baby had been picked up by the newspapers. A Rhode Island obstetrician, who had read the account and was clearly fasci-nated, came over to meet Ina May in Warwick, a small town near Providence, where the caravan was parked.

'He taught me everything that he could about emergency childbirth – what to do if the mother haemorrhaged, and how to give an injec-tion without injuring the mother. He was a kind man, and immensely popular, the sort of obstetrician that did what women wanted, and the consequence was that women wanted him to attend their births.' He also gave Ina May a copy of *The Handbook of Obstetrics and Gynecol-ogy* by Ralph Benson, a standard medical text that she found invaluable.

As Ina May went on to describe some of the highlights of the more than a thousand births she had attended over the past twenty years – difficulties encountered, and how she and her supporting team of some dozen newly recruited midwives coped – I was struck with the thought that the meeting with the Rhode Island OB must have laid the groundwork for Ina May's continuing, and often mutually beneficial, relationship with the medical/obstetrical profession. Unlike many midwives, who instinctively recoil at professionally trained doctors as hostile to their philosophy, Ina May is remarkably flexible, highly capable of both learning from and teaching members of the medical fraternity.

Soon after arriving at the Farm, Ina May had the great good fortune to fall in with yet another sympathetic physician, Dr John Williams, a general practitioner in Mount Pleasant, a fifteen-minute drive from the Farm. The nature-loving hippies had gathered a quantity of delicious watercress from a creek which, it turned out, was polluted by sewage. About a hundred people, a third of the whole population, became terribly ill with infectious hepatitis; although there were no fatalities, the hepatitis caused some premature births.

There were no telephones at the Farm (antithetical, perhaps, to the back-to-nature life-style?), so Ina May drove seven miles to the nearest pay phone and called Dr Williams, whom she had never met. She explained, 'I've got a woman in labour, guaranteed two months early. The baby is really tiny. What do I do?' Dr Williams, already sounding like everyone's personification of the good old-fashioned country doctor, told her to go ahead and deliver the baby. 'And then if it's small, just bring it right into town. I'll be in my office.'

The baby weighed two pounds, ten ounces. They wrapped it up warmly and drove to Mount Pleasant. 'Dr Williams took the tiny little thing in one hand, and he said: "Oh she looks like a good one." I liked the way he was so confident about it, and, you know, "Hi, darling!" to the mother.'

Thereafter Dr Williams became a fixture in the Farm's ever-growing midwifery practice. As Ina May told us, 'One thing I always treasure about him is that he never, ever got angry or cross if I called him up in the middle of the night. Pamela, one of our midwives, called him up once and said, "There's something blue coming out." He said, "Well, can you describe it, honey?" He would always be very fatherly like that. She said "Well, it's blue and shiny." We didn't have the medical terminology, not even anatomy. So he got in his pick-up truck, drove on out, and he says, "Oh, that's her cervix." He got a sterile glove, pushed it back, and out pops the baby's head, and then we learned, oh, you're supposed to do that.'

These hair-raising anecdotes might seem to substantiate the mainstream obstetricians' view that lay midwives are an ignorant, giddy lot whose ineptitude may endanger mother and child. While this might have been true in the early days of the Farm, there was the Dr Williams factor to make a big difference; not only did he make himself always available in an emergency, he freely shared his professional training, augmented by years of practical experience.

Ina May is at her best describing problem births and how she learned to deal with them. As the Farm women are mostly young, healthy, non-smokers, non-drinkers and non-druggers, they are on the whole unlikely to fall victim to the causes responsible for the soaring infant death rates in the rest of the country: lack of prenatal care, malnourishment, low birth weight.

If the expectant mother is suffering from a malady that puts her in the high-risk category such as diabetes or heart disease, the Farm midwives arrange to transfer her to Dr Williams's hospital for the birth.

At the Farm, as elsewhere, difficulties arise when the baby, which normally comes out head first, is in the wrong position – for example, breech (buttocks first), footling (a sweetly poetic designation, I thought, which means feet first), and worst of all transverse, in which the baby lies horizontally and can never emerge, no matter how long and arduous the labour.

In hospital, most of these would automatically be considered high-risk and would signal the call for an immediate Caesarean; but midwives have long been adept at 'version', manipulating the unborn externally by placing hands on the mother's abdomen and pushing and turning the infant until it is in its proper head-first position. And even if version doesn't work, the Farm midwives can with patience, encouragement, much oiling of the vaginal aperture and reaching with their hands to help the baby down, successfully manage these difficult deliveries.

Spiritual Midwifery, first produced in 1975 on the Farm's own printing press, gave detailed instructions in such matters in its lengthy technical section. It became an instant best-seller – 80,000 copies in the early editions, and well over half a million in several subsequent revisions. Ina May got letters from around the world: 'Somebody in Crete delivered a baby in a cave using my instructions, and another in a log cabin in Alaska,' she told me. 'It was all word of mouth, no advertising. Just the constant stream of visitors to the Farm, and some newspaper stories.'

Soon she was on her way to becoming an international celebrity in childbirth circles, in demand as a lecturer all over the United States and in a dozen European countries. Interestingly, these speaking engagements were by no means confined to the fairly circumscribed world of midwifery, but more and more included appearances at mainstream university medical schools and sessions with students of obstetrics.

At the time of our visit, Ina May had just been involved in a fracas over how to proceed in a case of 'shoulder dystocia', in plain English a stuck shoulder – the baby's head had emerged, but its shoulder was trapped behind the mother's pubic bone.

What to do? Ina May showed us directions set forth in *Nurse-Midwifery*, second edition, by Helen Varney, which says that the woman should be turned in bed on her side, and if this doesn't succeed she should be helped into a knee-chest position on the bed.

Ina May was appalled. This extremely influential text, required reading by all nurse-midwifery students and used by a good number of direct-entry midwives, is dead wrong, she said. 'Knee-chest is used if you want to slow down labour. And gravity alone would make the delivery almost impossible in that position.' Her solution, learned from Mayan midwives in the highlands of Guatemala, is to have the mother on all fours 'where her back is humped up, something like a cat, stretching. Then you've got a very favourable position for the stuck shoulders.'

After a lunch of tofu baked in a crust (no salt, deemed by Farm dwellers to be unhealthy – I murmured about the salt riots of the Middle Ages, to no avail), we repaired to a small studio off the living room to watch some of these achievements on video-cassettes, Farm-produced but of professional quality. There, in glorious Technicolor, with running voice-over commentary, were a breech birth followed by a stuck shoulder, both delivered vaginally. We saw the techniques described by Ina May being used in actual practice. It was a marvellous movie; Ted and I watched, riveted, and Betty Corbett's large blue eyes became as big as saucers – doubtless seeing herself in the role of a breech or stuck shoulder mother when her time came, just a few months off. The videotapes, we were told, are now widely used in some of the more up-and-coming medical school obstetrical courses.

During our discussions, it occurred to me that if Ina May had been plying her trade in medieval Europe she would have been a prime candidate for the stake, as she does have some distinctly witch-like attributes – such as ESP, second sight, and intuition. 'When a Farm member was close to having her baby, I would often find myself cutting my fingernails and the telephone would ring right then.' (Short, clean fingernails are for obvious reasons *de rigueur* for the midwife.) Nor would Ina May have been welcomed – or even tolerated – in nineteenth-century England. Part of her stock-in-trade is encouragement of sexual arousal of the woman in labour, achieved by the father's hugging, stroking, kissing – what Ida May inelegantly calls 'smooching'. This, she says, loosens up the cervix and thus makes for an easier, less painful, more enjoyable and speedier birth.

I was forcibly reminded of a stern warning by W. Tyler Smith in his 1847 article entitled 'On the Utility and Safety of the Inhalation of Ether in Obstetrical Practice':

> In many of the lower animals, we know that an erotic condition of the ovaria is present during parturition, and that sexual congress may take place immediately upon delivery. It was, however, reserved for the phenomenon of etherization to show that, as regards sexual emotion, the human female may possibly exchange the pangs of travail for the sensations of coitus, and so approach to the level of the brute creation.

Whether one is for or against exchanging the pangs of travail for the sensations of coitus (an idea that I must admit never occurred to me, nor can I imagine it happening with or without Ina May or 'etherization'), the really pertinent question is: What have been the success and failure rates of the Farm's midwifery practice?

The statistics as of 1989 are extremely reassuring: 1,700 births – 1.5 per cent Caesareans; 4.8 per cent transported to the hospital; 0.5 per cent forceps.

Farm midwives don't limit their practice to Farm dwellers, or visitors who come for the purpose of giving birth there. They also serve a large nearby community of Amish people, to whom they were recommended by Dr Williams. The Amish religion prohibits them from going to a hospital or otherwise participating in government-supported endeavours.

Thus the Farm midwifery clientele is a virtually all-white proposition, as are the clienteles of most latter-day home-birth midwives. For a dramatic change of venue, I sought out the Childbearing Center of Morris Heights, in the South Bronx.

Chapter 13

THE CHILDBEARING CENTER OF
MORRIS HEIGHTS

Dotted around the country are scores of 'freestanding' or 'alternative' birth centres, organised to provide maternity care for low-risk women who want to avoid the impersonal, sterile atmosphere of the hospital. According to a report from the National Association of Childbearing Centers in the *New England Journal of Medicine* (December 28, 1989), about twenty thousand babies have been born in the centres. Patients are typically white, middle-class, over eighteen, married, college-educated, well nourished. 'Almost all the women had adequate diets during pregnancy,' says the report. The centres are staffed by certified nurse-midwives, with a back-up obstetrician who will arrange transfer to a hospital in case of trouble. The cost, including regular prenatal care, postnatal visits and two consultations with the obstetrician, is about half that of a normal hospital delivery.

For a study in contrasts, in 1991 I turned to the Childbearing Center of Morris Heights in the South Bronx. Unique in the spectrum of freestanding birth centres, this is the only one in America established for the specific purpose of serving a poor, inner-city population. Jennifer Dohrn, director of the centre, described the neighbourhood: 'In this community forty per cent of the people live below the poverty level. It's about forty-five per cent black; a large number of Caribbeans; a growing African population. It's about forty-five per cent Latino, mainly Puerto Rican and Dominican, with a growing Central American population. It's also one of the centres for resettlement of Vietnam refugees.

'It's a community in crisis, ridden by crime, drugs, fighting to survive. Before we opened this birthing centre, one out of three women arrived at our back-up hospital, Bronx-Lebanon, in labour with no prenatal care. And our interpretation of this was not that women didn't care about having healthy babies, it was that they had been shut out of the system. There really was no access to getting prenatal care. To have to go and sit in the hospital for eight hours with small children, to see a different care provider for two minutes at each visit, to be told nothing about what's happening – this is not care that makes sense to anyone, nor is it feasible when mere survival is a daily struggle.'

When the centre first opened its doors on August 1, 1988, Jennifer Dohrn and her fellow midwives met with opposition not only from the medical fraternity but from many of the very people the centre was designed to serve, residents of Morris Heights.

'There was great scepticism in the medical community,' Jennifer said. 'Obstetricians said it made no sense for us to open a birthing centre in the South Bronx because anyone who lived here would be by definition "high-risk". Just living in poverty over the years would make a woman high-risk in terms of a normal pregnancy and birth.

'We, of course, did not believe this, and with the Manhattan Maternity Center Association, I was asked to build this birthing centre, and I'm doing it in conjunction with a local federally funded health-care clinic, the Morris Heights Health Care Center, which provides primary health care to this community.'

Another source of opposition to the centre was the older women, especially grandmothers who were recent immigrants. 'Their idea was that now they've come to the United States, and in particular New York City, their daughters should have the best birth possible – meaning in a hospital, because technology was a sign of progress. So we found a great resistance from many of these women until we began bringing them into the centre and explaining that we actually were combining the best of midwifery care and obstetrical care, that this was high-quality care. Now they are our advocates.'

The first objective of Jennifer and her co-workers was to spread the message. They visited every day-care centre, PTA, school, and health-care facility for miles around, bringing a slide show about birth, often accompanied by mothers whose babies had been born at the centre. 'We held brunches for grandmothers, dinners for fathers, but our biggest assets were the women who were attending prenatal sessions or had given birth in the centre. I realised that what we had here was the makings of a women's group. And with some support, with cooking some meals, with giving a bit of structure, with the work of a great outreach organiser, we have created a wonderful women's support group in this centre. They have formed a Community Action Committee, which is our main advisory group and really directs the life of the centre. They hold monthly meetings and are open to any woman who is pregnant, or if you've already had your baby, we'll cook a huge meal and the women will have picked topics to discuss from AIDS, to raising children, to breast-feeding. I often feel that we simply opened the door to the birthing centre and the women in this community made it their own.'

A major breakthrough came on February 19, 1989, with publication in the *Daily News*, the most widely read newspaper in the area, of an article by Heidi Evans, who had spent a day at the centre on call with Jennifer and had followed her through a birth. 'After her visit, she said, "I'll see that your centre never closes its doors,"' Jennifer recalled. 'Within a month of the article's appearance, enrolment in the centre jumped from thirty to ninety families, and we've been rolling ever since.'

What about financing, staff, number of births per year, and capacity – the nuts and bolts of the centre's operation?

'We had an original start-up grant of about eight hundred thousand dollars from the Kellogg Foundation – the cornflakes people, who spend millions on child health issues,' Jennifer said. Only about 15 to 20 per cent of the centre's clients have private health coverage; 50 per cent are on Medicaid. In between are the uninsured, women who don't qualify for Medicaid because somebody in the family is working. For these, there is a New York State programme called PCAP (Pregnancy Care Access Program) that covers the cost of care for pregnant women.

The centre is fortunate in having the services of administrative assistants who have mastered the art of propitiating the gods of bureaucracy. 'Anyone who comes in with no Medicaid and no private insurance immediately meets with one of them; she's very good at getting them on PCAP. She knows how to help people, and thanks to her work we are getting reimbursed for almost everyone who comes through here.' Medicaid now reimburses to the tune of $3,250 from the beginning of prenatal care through six weeks postpartum. This means, Jennifer said, that 'if every person who comes to the centre is on Medicaid, we can become financially self-sufficient. This is very unusual and very great.'

Yet another service offered by the centre is help in obtaining benefits from the Special Supplemental Feeding Program for Women, Infants, and Children (WIC), a federal programme for pregnant women, new mothers, and children up to the age of five. WIC supplies basic foods such as infant formula, milk, cereal, juice, eggs, dried beans, and peanut butter. To qualify, a woman must produce an application signed by her health provider giving details of her pregnancy – due date, hematocrit (a blood test for anaemia), other minutiae such as whether the mother is younger than nineteen, or has had two babies within a year – as well as documentation of her financial status, such as rent receipts. The application is daunting for a new immigrant or a high-school dropout, 'but we have made the process easier by having a WIC representative in our centre. WIC also provides us with a nutritionist three hours per week,' Jennifer told me.

What of the regular centre staff – categories and wages? I asked Jennifer. She gave me a breakdown:

Four midwives, three white, one black. As of autumn 1991, their salaries ranged from $45,000 to $50,000.

Five midwife assistants, three Latinas, two blacks, and all local residents; salaries $15,000.

One project administrator, Nigerian, the only man on the professional staff.

One receptionist, one janitor.

An obstetrician, Indian, who comes for a three-hour session once a week in which all cases are reviewed – approximately $200 a session.

Two social workers, one white and one Puerto Rican.

These last two are invaluable, Jennifer said. 'Life in the South Bronx is all about sheer survival – a mother has no food for her family of six, or maybe is a victim of battering. The social workers can be of tremendous help in such circumstances.'

Recruiting professional staff is very difficult, Jennifer said, as they could earn much more in a big city hospital; salaries have been a struggle. Midwives' salaries have more than doubled in New York in five years; from 1986 to 1991 they have risen from $30,000 to $65,000 or $70,000 in a private hospital. 'Any one of us could go out and make ten to fifteen thousand dollars more. And conditions of work in the South Bronx are deplorable; it's a dangerous community, and we work long hours. A night worker may get ready to go home in the morning only to find that her car has been stolen.

'In the three and a half years since we've been open [as of late 1991], the centre has proved to be so successful that the Health and Hospitals Corporation of New York City now has a plan to open two birthing centres next year,' Jennifer said. 'I think we'll be a model.'

A friend whom I'll call CR, herself a registered nurse with wide experience in big public hospitals in Detroit, Atlanta, and New York City, spent a day in October 1991 visiting the Morris Heights Center, touring the premises, and interviewing the personnel. She wrote to me:

At 9:00 a.m. I reached Jennifer Dohrn on the phone. 'I'm with a mom, pushing,' she said. 'Push on,' said I, 'I'll be there shortly.'

The center is located in a small building across the street from the Morris Heights Health Center. The outer door is locked, and entry is gained by being buzzed in. The front door is covered with pink and blue slips announcing the names, dates, and birthweights of recent arrivals. Upon entering, one immediately senses a warm and comfortable atmosphere; the receptionist, Ethel Gittens,

a young black woman, is full of smiles and greetings. The waiting area is furnished with cozy couches and tables with current
magazines and health educational materials. A janitor is lov-
ingly attending to a huge tub of plants in the center of the room.
One wall is taken up by rows of paper plaques, each inscribed with
the name of a center-born baby.

Jennifer comes down dressed in blue scrubs carrying the newborn baby girl, minutes old, daughter of a fourteen-year-old girl.
The seven-pound, three-ounce baby appears purple, wrinkled and
waterlogged like all newborns, making fish-mouth faces, fists
clenched. Ethel Gittens happily announces the news of the birth
on the telephone.

Soon, the newly delivered mother and baby are resting, while
the teenager's grandmother, with whom she lives, is in the kitchen
preparing some food. The baby's father is restlessly walking about,
looking scared and proud.

The center is a lovely combination of informal home-like rooms
with all the elements needed to run a health care business. There
are several offices, a meeting room, two examination rooms for
expectant mothers in prenatal care, and a play room for their kids
who are always welcome. There is a fully equipped kitchen where
family members can prepare their own food if they prefer, or eat
food provided by the center. There's a dining room with chairs, a
couch and television set.

The two delivery rooms resemble home bedrooms with curtains,
bedspreads, and pictures, all colorful and non-institutional. The
beds are firm, and have been raised a few inches for the sake of
the midwives' backs.

Clinic hours begin at noon, and the waiting area is gradually
filling up with expectant mothers and their young children, bust-
ling about and chatting.

A near-term woman who has been experiencing a lot of discomfort for the past week is examined. It is determined that she
is not in labor, so she is given reassurance and instructions before
returning home. Another woman comes in after her waters broke
at home. She is not in labor. Jennifer explains that they will try to
bring on labor within twelve hours by having the woman drink

castor oil*. If this doesn't work, she will have to go to the hospital. All these activities take place in a calm, unhurried, unharried atmosphere. The attention given each woman is personal, caring, and professionally competent.

Later, wandering through the building, I talked with some of the people who have made this center what it is today.

Ethel Gittens, the receptionist who establishes the tone of the place when one first steps inside, has been here for three and a half years, since the beginning, having worked previously at the Manhattan Maternity Center Association. I asked why women come here, rather than go to a hospital. At first, there were many dropouts, she said: 'Women would register, and then their mothers would encourage them to go to the hospital when they went into labor. The parents or husbands would get nervous, even though the young women themselves seemed quite comfortable with us. We have lots of teenagers here – there's a special teen parent program for these.'

Dana Keys, a black mother whose fifth baby was born here in April 1991, described the birth of her third child in North Central Bronx Hospital, which she chose because they have a midwife program there. 'There is a midwife to deliver the baby, but there's also a doctor. Doctors don't have the patience that midwives have. The baby was not coming forth due to a large head, so the doctor wanted to give me a cesarean. The midwives were saying let's wait, and I was saying the same thing. But the doctor said he was going to get a court order, and while he was in the process of doing this, the baby was born. It was a very uncomfortable experience, I was tense, although the midwife was there and she did her best to help me and keep me calm.'

She learned about the center from a newspaper article, made an appointment for a tour of the facilities, immediately signed up for

---

* Castor oil, unheard of by me as a remedy to bring on labour, evokes memories. When I was a girl in the 1930s, the prescription in England for a self-induced miscarriage was lots of castor oil, lots of quinine, lots of gin, and lie in a very hot bath until you faint. I am not sure if it worked, or if many drowned in the hot bath, but some of my contemporaries thought it an excellent recipe in days when abortions were illegal.

what she described as the best birth of her five children: 'It's a place where you feel secure. And not just having a baby – family planning, discussion of personal problems. The midwives and clients become personal friends. You stop by to visit long after the baby's born. It's a fabulous place. It's more than just a place to have a baby. These people become part of your life – it's an ongoing thing. You see women coming in who've had their babies here and now the babies are walking. They come in to talk.'

The on-the-job training for midwife assistants was described by Hilda Alvarez, who has served in this capacity for three years: 'Before that, I was a housewife. I never did any work with patient care before. I live in this neighborhood, a fifteen-minute walk. We have to see five births, to watch everything so we can hand the midwives anything they need. When the baby is about to be born we get oxygen for the baby or the suction machine if needed. We give the mother a back rub and a hot blanket. You keep training as you work.'

As word of the center spread, women from other communities around New York started to come for prenatal care and birth. Zakiyyah Madyun was living on 168th Street when at the age of thirty-nine she had her first baby, in the center, having found the address in the Yellow Pages. 'I knew from the moment when I walked in the door that I was home. The atmosphere – I was able to identify as an African-American woman; there wasn't anything like a hospital about it. You actually feel like you walked into your own home when you come in here.' She is now working as residency coordinator in the Bronx-Lebanon Department of Family Practice, is secretary of the Community Action Committee, and member of the Breastfeeding Council. She has gone around the country representing the center. Asked how she would describe this community, she said, 'That's a very touchy question. There are many fallacies about indigent communities, and one of them is the assumption that if you come from a medically indigent area you lack intelligence. You lack initiative, you're probably on drugs, you have multiple sex partners – these are all ideas that are attached to people who live in these kinds of communities.' The visual aspects play into these prejudices, she said: '"Why don't they keep up their streets? Pick up their garbage?" When the fact is that the city officials don't maintain our neighborhoods like they do other areas in the Bronx or Manhattan.'

What propelled Jennifer Dohrn into this arduous job? First, a general disgust with what she described as 'the culture of birth in this society. Things are done to us. We are delivered of our babies, as opposed to us ourselves birthing our babies. And this is considered, quote, the best way to have a baby, the safest way. Of course it's all very tied into economics and the building of modern obstetrics and the whole medical profession into a large corporate business. There's also a very strong tie-in with the oppression of women.'

And why, in particular, was she drawn to Morris Heights? 'I have a real particular passion – mission – calling – to try and direct attention not only to what is happening to childbirth in this country, but also to draw attention to what's happening to poor women, and that means especially women of colour, in childbirth, because for every crime in terms of their treatment in childbirth that's been committed against women in the middle or upper class, it's so many more times severe for women who have no money, often a language barrier, and who are also subject to the racism of this society.'

Chapter 14

MIDWIVES UNDER THE GUN

A funny thing happened to Patricia Craig in July 1990 as she was leaving to teach her regular class at the Sage Femme Midwifery School in La Selva, California, of which she was the director. She was presented with an affidavit – 'Sign this, or else!' – prepared by one Katherine Blakeney, investigator for the California Board of Medical Quality Assurance. The affidavit, on the letterhead of the California State Department of Consumer Affairs, declared 'under penalty of perjury': 'I am no longer the Director or an instructor, or in any way affiliated with the Sage Femme Midwifery School, which is no longer in existence.' There followed a lengthy quotation from Section 2052 of the California Business and Professions Code, which makes it a misdemeanour to practise medicine without a licence. The affidavit continued:

> I am aware that the unlawful practice of medicine which results in the injury of any person may be a felony under Section 2053 of the California Business and Professions Code, and that aiding or abetting the unlicensed practice of medicine is also a violation of the law. I will not participate, encourage, or give any instruction in lay midwifery in the future.

As background: Patricia Craig had served as a lay, or direct-entry, midwife in the Santa Cruz area and San Francisco County for ten years, during which time she had assisted at more than 150 home births with outstanding success, attested to in a stack of letters from satisfied customers. She had never had what is called in obstetrical jargon a 'bad outcome', meaning a dead or damaged baby or an injured mother. No complaints had ever been filed against her.

For the past three years, Ms Craig had been director and teacher at the Sage Femme Midwifery School, whose objectives were to educate aspirant midwives in the skills of that calling and to prepare them to qualify for the California Association of Midwives (CAM) certification programme. Sage Femme's printed brochure specifically stated that 'completion of the course does not confer an accredited degree', and it contained a legal disclaimer: 'Graduation from Sage Femme Midwifery School, or a certification with the California Association of Midwives, does not confer a license to practice midwifery within the state of California.'

The CAM certification programme is an effort to lay to rest, once and for all, the allegation of 'practicing medicine without a license'. To qualify, the prospective midwife must complete a rigorous academic course of study such as that offered by Sage Femme – plus practical 'hands-on' experience as apprentice to a midwife.

The end goal is for midwives to become self-certified and self-policing through stringent peer review, and eventually to achieve legislative recognition as professionals in their field – much as other unorthodox health practitioners, such as acupuncturists and chiropractors, achieved legal status in California.

'But wherein lies the crime of Patricia Craig?' the puzzled reader may wonder. 'Is midwifery illegal, and if so, why?'

The laws governing the practice of direct-entry midwives vary wildly from state to state. The American College of Obstetricians and Gynecologists 'Fifty State Comprehensive Survey' of 1986, covering both certified nurse-midwives and lay midwives, gave a concise summary. In New Mexico, for example, a lay midwife – who must pass stiff requirements for certification – is not only legally authorised to practise home births for low-risk women, but is entitled to mandatory third-party reimbursement by health insurance plans. In Texas, the lay midwife is permitted to practise but required to inform her client of the 'limitations of her skills and practices'. In Oregon, no laws prohibit the practice of lay midwifery. In Pennsylvania and Ohio the practice of lay midwifery is prohibited by law. In between are many states in which the law is ambiguous.

And what of California? The ACOG survey merely stated, 'There are currently no statutory or regulatory provisions governing the practice of lay midwifery in California.'

Maybe yes, maybe no, depending on who's telling it. The confusion arises from an old law on the books authorising non-nurse midwives to attend births. However, the licensing provisions of this law were revoked in 1949. After that date, no new lay midwives could be licensed, although renewal of licences already held was permitted. Several old-timers continued to renew their licences under this statute until fairly recently, when the last of them died. Hence the anomaly: a licensed lay midwife can practise, but there is no mechanism for obtaining a licence. Catch-22. That's why California midwives are seeking new legislation under which they can be licensed.

Enter BMQA, the Board of Medical Quality Assurance (which in 1991 recently changed its name to the less euphonious Medical Board of California).

This agency, operating under the umbrella of the Department of Consumer Affairs, is charged with licensing physicians and policing the profession for the protection of the public, with authority to suspend or revoke the licence of incompetents and other bad actors. A majority of the board members are practising physicians, nominated by their local medical societies. The board employs about forty investigators statewide.

Of recent years, BMQA has devoted much energy to the harassment of home-birth midwives. Why the implacable hostility of the medical establishment to their practice? A possible answer, as Deep Throat told Woodward and Bernstein in the dark recesses of that sinister garage: 'Follow the money.'

A highly regarded Berkeley obstetrician told me in 1990 that for a normal vaginal delivery his seven-member medical group charges $2,365; for a Caesarean, the fee goes up to $3,220, to which must be added, of course, the ever-escalating hospital bills. In the San Francisco Bay area a midwife's fee for prenatal care, attendance at birth, and subsequent house calls runs to about $900 to $1,200. As the majority of home-birth clients are middle-class women with ample insurance for whom cost is not a major consideration, the midwives believe that the medical community's vendetta against them is to a large extent motivated by fear of losing paying clients.

Aside from its efforts to stamp out home-birth midwifery, what was BMQA doing to protect the public? Not much, it seems.

In April 1989, the Center for Public Interest Law in San Diego issued a devastating 100-page report entitled 'Physician Discipline in California: A Code Blue Emergency' (Code Blue being the hospital term for a life-threatening situation), in which it stated that 'Physician discipline in California ... cannot and does not protect Californians from incompetent medical practice. It is effectively moribund.'

Its principal findings: 'Each year the Medical Board receives upwards of 20,000 calls from consumers about physicians. It considers about 6,000 of those serious enough to categorise as a complaint. Typically over 5,800 of those are dismissed or taken care of informally, sometimes through a verbal admonition from Board staff or a member of one of the Board's regional enforcement committees.'

On further whittling down, the report states that 'a grand total of twelve physicians were subject to *any* discipline (revocation, suspension, or probation) in 1987–88 for incompetence, and five for abuse of drugs or alcohol. These levels are typical, not aberrational statistics.'

BMQA fought back through the pages of *California Physician*, the slick monthly magazine of the California Medical Association. The rebuttal, which took up most of the June 1989 issue, was surprisingly wimpish. Aside from castigating the report by the Center for Public Interest Law as 'purple rhetoric' and 'a clear attempt to panic the public', the CMA analysis had nothing much to offer in BMQA's defence.

In a separate article BMQA director Kenneth Wagstaff seemed to agree with most of the recommendations by the Center for Public Interest Law, 'some of which are from BMQA', and, like a good bureaucrat, saw it as confirming the need for more money for more staff to tackle the backlog of complaints.

Wishing to get the facts from the horse's mouth, so to speak, I sought a meeting with Mr Wagstaff at BMQA's Sacramento headquarters on August 22, 1989.

My objectives were simple: to elucidate further BMQA's response to the report by the Center for Public Interest Law and to discover why, in view of BMQA's admittedly huge backlog of consumer complaints against physicians, its investigators would spend such an inordinate amount of time pursuing midwives, against whom there has been *no* complaint from the families they serve.

What about the finding by the Center for Public Interest Law that in 1987–88 only 12 physicians out of 71,000 practising in California were subject to *any* discipline for incompetence?

Mr Wagstaff: 'To say that only twelve formal disciplines for incompetence in one year accurately reflects the impact of the board on physician practice is akin to saying that the only impact the California Highway Patrol has on drivers is reflected in the number of convictions for drunk driving.'

This seemed like odd reasoning, particularly in view of the trial of Dr Milos Klvana then in progress in Los Angeles for the deaths of eight babies and a foetus. Klvana's activities had been unhampered by BMQA, which allowed him to continue practising for ten years after his initial conviction on twenty-six criminal counts of illegally prescribing controlled substances – and for eight years after the first infant death was reported to BMQA.

At the time of my interview with Wagstaff, Dr Klvana's trial for murder had been going on for five months. I don't know how the Highway Patrol would have handled this case, but Mr Wagstaff was more than a little hazy about the facts.

J. M.: 'Let me ask you, have you ever heard of the case of Dr Milos Klvana?'

Wagstaff: 'Yes, I have. I don't know what – yes, I remember – what do I know about Klvana? I don't remember very well.'

At this point, Linda McCready, BMQA's external affairs coordinator and Mr Wagstaff's chief mouthpiece, came to his rescue, saying Klvana had 'a number of unfortunate outcomes that we believe may have involved negligence or incompetence. He was convicted, as I recall.'

Not so, I pointed out; he was still on trial for the murder of eight babies. Going through the record, in 1980 BMQA had placed Klvana on five years' probation, meaning that he was still free to practise. In 1982, one baby died. In 1983, BMQA lifted Klvana's probation.

Two more babies died. BMQA took no action. In 1984, three babies died. The Los Angeles district attorney's office took over the case. In 1985, a baby died. In 1986, a baby died; Klvana was arrested and charged with second-degree murder. In 1987, out on bail, Klvana resumed practice. In 1988, his bail was revoked. Klvana was back in jail. At this point, BMQA revoked his licence.

His memory jogged, Mr Wagstaff replied, 'The guy had marvellous attorneys ... It's been a while since I thought much about Klvana ... it's hard to deal with an individual case.'

J. M.: 'You wouldn't let a guy run around killing people that long before you did something about it?'

Wagstaff: 'The question is like when did I stop beating my wife.'

Alas for BMQA. The question persisted – and escalated to a huge furor after Dr Klvana was convicted in December 1989. The ten-month trial ended on December 18, three months after my interview with Mr Wagstaff. The Los Angeles jury found the doctor guilty of nine counts of second-degree murder (eight infants and a foetus), as well as numerous lesser counts.

At this point, possibly jolted by the verdicts, BMQA lumbered into action and conducted a hastily organised 'internal investigation' of its handling of the Klvana case. Seldom can what political pundits call 'damage control' have backfired more disastrously on the would-be controllers.

On February 5, three days after the results of the internal investigation had appeared in the newspapers, Los Angeles Superior Court Judge Judith Chirlin sentenced the doctor to a 53-years-to-life prison term. In a rare display of courtroom unanimity among the frequently warring elements in a criminal trial, defence, prosecutor, judge, and jury all tore into BMQA for its negligence:

Deputy District Attorney Brian R. Kelberg, prosecutor: 'I hope the court will make some statements about the medical board of California. They have a lot of lambasting that should be forthcoming to them, and I hope this court will take the opportunity.'

Richard A. Leonard, defence attorney: 'They should have taken away his licence and saved a few babies' lives ... They took his word as the whole truth. They should have known he had a motive to lie to them to save his licence. They should have done a better job investigating the case.'

Jury foreman Jaime Pulido and juror Sam Orr: The two jurors fired off a six-page 'open letter' to Mr Wagstaff and California legislators in which they declared that 'the sham self-policing procedures that made Dr Klvana possible are still in place and the Medical Board of California continues to fight efforts to tighten those procedures . . . in fact, we find the medical board's performance so irresponsible that we wish there were a way for them to share in the verdicts.'

Judge Judith Chirlin: Pronouncing sentence on Dr Klvana, Judge Chirlin delivered a scorching rebuke to BMQA:

> And this is the board that we have to protect us against unscrupulous and incompetent doctors?
>
> One can imagine, and I hope share, the outrage that I felt when reading in *The Los Angeles Times* on Friday, February 2, 1990, that an 'internal inquiry into how state medical authorities handled an investigation of Milos Klvana found no need for major institutional reforms'. The chairman of the board's medical quality division was quoted as saying, 'Overall, I would say the system is adequate.'
>
> To me it looks like the board did an even worse job investigating itself than it did in investigating Dr Klvana.
>
> How many more dead babies or dead patients of other incompetent doctors will it take before the BMQA is forced to take a serious and in-depth look at its procedures?

And now for an update.

Apparently these furious comments by the judge and the comments of other outraged trial participants have had absolutely no effect on the conduct of the medical board. On February 16, 1992, three years after the Klvana trial, *The San Francisco Examiner* ran a front page story by Tupper Hall of the newspaper's Sacramento bureau. He wrote:

> A San Diego doctor is charged with raping five patients based in part on complaints, some going back to 1983, filed with the state board in charge of policing physician conduct, but never acted on.

Hall went on to elaborate:

The California Medical Board [formerly BMQA] is taking an average of 2.8 years to investigate, prosecute and resolve cases, according to the state auditor general.

Those figures include cases in which the accused doctors do not fight their discipline.

When the doctors fight and take their appeals to the state courts, discipline against errant physicians commonly takes six to eight years to resolve, according to University of San Diego law professor Robert Fellmeth, one of the state's foremost experts on the state's regulatory authority.

'During this interim, in virtually every case, the physician maintains his or her license in good standing and is free to practice medicine within the state of California,' Fellmeth said.

'In short, the system is a mess. It is mired in an "old boys club" mentality. It is fragmented, clogged, slow, embarrassingly solicitous of the profession, and produces virtually nothing.'

At a meeting in Santa Cruz on June 1, 1989, with a dozen practising direct-entry midwives and certified nurse-midwives, I got a strong whiff of BMQA's methods and its capacity for striking terror into the subjects of surveillance. The BMQA tactics were strangely reminiscent of those of the FBI at the height of the McCarthy witch-hunt in the mid-1950s. Some comments from the group:

'The harassment has been increasing in the last couple of years. Midwives come home to find the card of the local BMQA agent pinned on their door, and that's that.'

'And then she'll find out secondhand that all of her previous clients have been telephoned by the agent, although she hasn't been questioned.'

'She may have kids at home, she doesn't want to go to jail so she gets paranoid, cleans her whole house out, files and equipment – I've done it a few times, taken everything to a friend's house for safekeeping.'

'Midnight cleaning! Midnight cleaning! Frantic house cleaning . . .'

The speakers, mind you, were all women with long unblemished careers as home-birth midwives, with nary a complaint from the families they served. Listening to their accounts, I was forcibly reminded of a passage in the *Malleus Maleficarum*, the fifteenth-century rule book for the Inquisition:

> Her house should be searched as thoroughly as possible, in all holes and corners and chests, top and bottom; and if she is a noted witch, then without doubt, unless she has previously hidden them, there will be found various instruments of witchcraft, as we have shown above.

The only physician in the group, Dr Greg Troll, said BMQA's handling of complaints against doctors was 'very, very different. I worked for a doctor who was investigated for drug and alcohol abuse and it was all very polite. The investigators were respectful to him, none of this raiding of his home or seizure of his files. He was ushered into a "diversion" programme to be cured of his addiction, and that was the end of it.'

Not surprisingly, some midwives have caved in under the BMQA's systematic programme of intimidation; they have relinquished their practice or fled to more hospitable territory such as New Mexico, Oregon, or Texas.

One who fought back is Sally Wright, a midwife in Roseville, California. She described her truly bizarre experience with BMQA agents: she was at home with two of her three children on April 5, 1990, when at about 12:30 p.m. she heard loud banging on the front door and shouts of 'Open up! Police!' Before she could get to the door six men armed with pistols burst in. They ordered her and the children, aged five and eleven, to stay in the living room while they ransacked the house, for which they had a search warrant.

In scenes straight out of *The Twilight Zone*, the BMQA police were reinforced by two additional policemen. Ms Wright's third child, nine years old, arrived from school. The three children became hysterical; Ms Wright was not only under house arrest but under *room* arrest, not permitted to leave her living room to see what the BMQA agents were doing. Why? she asked. 'Because you might have a gun,' they replied. Some days later, BMQA spokesman Linda McCready, when asked why the investigators were armed, explained to the press,

'When you go into a home, you don't know what you are going to find. You are prepared for the worst.'

Again, the *Malleus Maleficarum* anticipates this procedure:

> If she be taken in her own house, let her not be given time to go into her room; for they are wont to secure in this way, and bring away with them, some object or power of witchcraft.

Ms Wright's request that she be allowed to phone her mother to come and get the children was first refused, then granted after the investigators got tired of the offstage sounds of screaming children. 'When my mother arrived, the BMQA investigators demanded to see her ID before "turning over" the children to her. I told them, "These are not your children, they are mine. This is my house."' She won that round; the children left with their grandmother, but thereafter have suffered recurrent nightmares about the events of April 5.

After three hours of searching, the BMQA team departed, carrying out thirty-eight boxes of Ms Wright's possessions – a strange miscellany that included not only a Doppler heart monitor (part of a midwife's necessary equipment) and patients' records, but books, magazines about child care, toilet articles, even a hair-curling iron. These items were all impounded and turned over to the district attorney as evidence of Ms Wright's practising medicine without a licence. I visualise some neophyte assistant district attorney sorting through the boxes, scratching his head and wondering what the devil those curling irons are used for. Possibly on a baby born with straight hair? And why is a book about the US Constitution evidence of a crime? It might take years to figure out the relevance of this assortment.

Five days after the raid, about a hundred of Sally Wright's friends and supporters, many of them families with children whose births she had attended, rallied to her defence at a very polite and muted demonstration at the state capitol – which nevertheless got considerable coverage by the Sacramento press and TV news. Channel 13 ran two call-in polls: Should home-birth midwifery be legalised? The 6:00 p.m. poll recorded 77 per cent in favour, 23 per cent opposed; the 11:00 p.m. poll, 82 per cent for, 18 per cent against.

Getting answers on the cases of Patricia Craig and Sally Wright was not easy. In August 1990, I called the office of Jack Shelley, district attorney in Roseville. His press secretary told me he wasn't sure whether Ms Wright would be prosecuted or the charges dropped: 'The case is under review.' When will her goods be returned to her? 'After the investigation is completed, probably some time in September.'

Back to Mr Wagstaff at BMQA, who also wasn't sure of anything about the Craig and Wright cases, although in answer to my question as to where he personally stands on the midwife issue he said, surprisingly, 'I wish the state legislature would make it legal.' He supports the California Association of Midwives effort for self-licensing and hopes the legislature will concur. About Patricia Craig – he hadn't seen the BMQA affidavit, so wasn't sure if the threat therein was a violation of the First Amendment; he hadn't seen the prospectus of the Sage Femme Midwifery School.

Wagstaff referred me to Ward Jayne, head of the San Mateo office and supervisor of Katherine Blakeney, who, he assured me, could answer all my questions. Could, maybe, but wouldn't, on the grounds that discussion of a case 'under investigation' is prohibited by the medical board's rules; and Jayne hung up.

Obfuscation plus. Vernon Leeper, BMQA's chief investigator in Sacramento, also wouldn't or couldn't discuss these matters, which are, he said, 'confidential'.

After days of my frustrating effort to breach these stone walls, Mr Wagstaff came through with a sort-of explanation of the medical board's sign-or-else affidavit thrust upon Patricia Craig. 'We do this in cases where legal action is not now contemplated, but where we wish to obtain confirmation that the subject of the investigation will cease activities which could lead to future action on our part.' He added that if Ms Craig should choose not to sign, 'we no doubt will do nothing further because her midwifery-school activities have ceased'. There were, he said, no charges against Craig apart from teaching.

In other words, the affidavit was merely an exercise in intimidation, its intent to scare Craig into closing her school; but it didn't work. Contrary to Mr Wagstaff's belief, her school is flourishing; she has more students than ever and is advertising her courses in the local press. Furthermore, if the medical board should be so foolhardy as to haul her into court, it would have the American Civil Liberties Union to contend with. The ACLU has pledged support and representation of Ms Craig and her teaching as protected by the First Amendment.

While in the case of the physician serial rapist the medical board 'remained in a wise and masterly inactivity' (as Sir James Mackintosh, an eighteenth-century British writer, said of the House of Commons), the board was unremitting in its zealous pursuit of midwives. Sixteen months after the raid by armed investigators on Sally Wright's home, a worse fate befell Faith Gibson, a Mennonite midwife of Palo Alto, California.

On August 9, 1991, her class on breast-feeding was rudely interrupted when medical board agents burst into her house, announced that she was under arrest, handcuffed her, and dragged her off to the county jail, known euphemistically, as such places are, as the 'Women's Correctional Facility'. In the event, the 'correction' was short-lived, as friends bailed her out within ten hours. There was a flurry of headlines in the Bay Area newspapers: 'Medical-legal Tempest Swirls About Calm Mennonite Midwife', San Jose *Mercury News*; 'State Battles Local Midwife', *San Francisco Chronicle*; 'Palo Alto Midwife Held on 4 Licensing Charges', *San Francisco Chronicle*.

The charges against 48-year-old Faith Gibson have an all too familiar ring: practising midwifery without a licence, practising nursing without a licence, advertising midwifery services without a licence, and advertising nursing services without a licence. Together, the four misdemeanour offences carry a penalty of a year in prison and a $1,000 fine. There was nothing in the charges to suggest that she had harmed any mothers or babies, and for good reason: in the past twenty years, she has attended over four thousand births, some as a hospital delivery room nurse, and as lay midwife she has presided over three hundred and fifty home births, with never a mishap.

How did the medical board investigators go about gathering evidence for the charges against Faith Gibson, given the impossibility of securing a complaint against her from any of her clients or their families? At first, the best they could come up with was a complaint from a disgruntled former landlady to the Board of Registered Nursing to the effect that Ms Gibson was running an illegal midwifery practice. Deeming this insufficient, the investigators – borrowing, perhaps, from higher-up dirty tricks role models in the CIA and FBI – devised their own super-sleuth methods. One can imagine them huddling together to discuss strategy.

The upshot: several covert operators visited Faith Gibson, one posing as a woman interested in home birth, another as a salesman whose wife was eight and a half months pregnant. They borrowed videotapes that showed Ms Gibson attending a home birth. She reckons that she received five or more entrapment calls between June and August; the last call was just two days before her arrest.

This may have been both pleasurable and remunerative for the undercover investigators; but it would be of more than passing interest if some whistle-blower in the medical board, or a consumer advocate with powers of subpoena, could add up the wages of the medical board operatives for the many hours they spent at taxpayers' expense on this patently absurd investigation.

Faith Gibson has the good fortune to be represented by some of the best legal talent in the state: Anne Flower Cumings, a distinguished lawyer who has represented many accused midwives; and Paul Halvonik, a nationally renowned constitutional lawyer.

Mr Halvonik came round to explain to me the issues as he sees them. He was a pleasure to watch, playing about with the California law governing lay midwifery (described on pages 187–8), worrying it like a terrier with a bone, finally reducing it to a pitiful heap of rubble.

Striding about the living room, he could have been declaiming to a judge and jury – note, for example, his repetition of the defendant's name, a common lawyerly device to 'humanise' the suspected criminal he is defending; and his use of unusual, attention-getting words such as 'unforehandedly' and 'irrebuttably':

'Faith Gibson is not charged with doing something that is, in itself, illegal. Midwifery is not illegal (so they say) in California. Faith Gibson is not charged with lacking the qualifications for a California midwife. Faith Gibson is not charged with performing poorly as a midwife. Faith Gibson is charged with not having a licence,' said Halvonik.

'At the same time, it is forbidden that she have a licence. California's midwife licence is available only as a renewal to one who possessed one in 1949. Faith was born in 1947 and, unforehandedly, made no application when she was two.

'Faith Gibson is challenging a law providing, flatly, that the only people competent to function as midwives are those who were honing their skills during the Truman administration. And yet, one does no dishonour to tradition by entertaining the possibility that, since 1949, someone has come along who can handle the task. A rule that no one who was not a judge or legislator in 1949 is irrebuttably incompetent to function in the capacity would, one suspects, attract constitutional objection.'

As of this writing, March 1992, the outcome of *People of the State of California v. Bonnie Faye Gibson* (for such was Faith's original name) is unknown. As in any criminal case, there are many options – the district attorney could dismiss for lack of evidence; the defendant could be acquitted; or she could be found guilty and appeal all the way to the Supreme Court. Months or years could go by before the case is resolved. In the meantime, lay midwives are as vulnerable as ever to the onslaughts of the medical board investigators.

However, as in all good Westerns, help is on the way in the shape of California State Senator Lucy Killea, who, at the behest of embattled midwives, came riding forth with a bill that would once and for all establish the direct-entry midwife as a fully licensed legal practitioner.

In September 1991, I went to part of a three-day conference of the California Association of Midwives (CAM) in Sacramento, the state capital. The turnout was large, about 250 direct-entry midwives and a goodly number of certified nurse-midwives, who say they have much to learn from the practical, hands-on experience of their direct-entry counterparts, much of which was missing from the medically prescribed courses they took in CNM training.

I skipped the many technical panels on topics such as 'Beginning Suturing', 'Advanced Suturing', 'Drawing Blood', and 'Haemorrhage', all doubtless of great interest to the midwives. I was after the presentations of Senator Lucy Killea and her extremely able legislative aide, Nancy Chavez. The whole point of the Killea bill is that it demolishes the opposition's argument that legalisation would open the door to anyone who has a sudden urge to try her hand at home delivery, no matter how inadequate her training or qualifications. On the contrary, as Senator Killea eloquently pointed out, her bill mandates a long training period before a licence can be granted, the specifics of which were developed and spelled out by the California Association of Midwives.

Long, loud cheers all around. Nancy Chavez explained the mechanics of campaigning – how to establish a grass-roots demand, how to enlist your own state senator or representative. More loud cheers, and pledges of active participation from the audience. It was an inspiriting occasion. But being inured, over a long life, to seeing good causes demolished by special-interest groups, I didn't expect much to come of this. So I was surprised and pleased when Senator Killea's bill was passed on July 15, 1991, by one of the toughest legislative watchdogs, the Senate Business and Professions Committee, on a vote of 5 to 1.

So far, so good – but too soon to declare victory, because in the next round, a hearing before the Senate Appropriations Committee, on January 13, 1992 the bill was killed by a 9 to 2 vote.

By then, the California Medical Association had mobilised its big guns. Although the California Nursing Association and the American College of Nurse-Midwives in an unprecedented show of solidarity with direct-entry midwives came to testify in support of the Killea bill, joined by many obstetricians, and physicians who broke with their professional societies, the money and power of the medical establishment won out – for the moment, but perhaps not for ever. In the spirit of *Destry Rides Again*, Senator Killea vowed to reintroduce her bill until it becomes law.

For me, one of the most interesting things about the medical opposition to this legislation arose out of my discussion in April 1990 with Dr Warren Pearse of the American College of Obstetricians and Gynecologists. In all our discussions and subsequent correspondence, Pearse came through as a firm supporter of certified nurse-midwives – and an equally dedicated opponent of the licensure of direct-entry midwives. Why so? I asked, having explained the proposed course of study for direct-entry midwives in California. 'These programmes need to be given in an institution of higher education, not by three ladies who think it's a nice idea,' he said.

Apart from the dreamed-up three nice ladies, suppose the programme should meet the standards of the World Health Organization? In that case, Pearse would be in favour of it. Nevertheless, his organisation and the whole powerful CMA came out against the Killea bill.

On January 16, 1992, the following appeared as the lead editorial in *The San Francisco Chronicle*:

A Good Idea: Midwife Delivery
The key to having healthy babies and healthy mothers in California is having competent, relatively inexpensive medical care available before, during and after the birth process. It is a real disgrace that the United States, with one of the most advanced medical systems in the world, ranks 22nd in terms of percentage of deaths in the first year of life.

In this state, 9 out of 1,000 babies die before their first birthday. One reason is that more than 7 percent of women delivering children have had no prenatal care. This lack of expert supervision takes a desperate toll.

State Senator Lucy Killea, D-San Diego, has proposed a thoughtful, constructive remedy in legislation that would legalize practice by midwives. The state currently allows specially trained nurses to give birth and prenatal care primarily in hospitals under direction of physicians. But some 40 years ago, the state stopped providing licenses to allow midwives to deliver babies at home.

Senator Killea's bill, SB 1190, was replete with safeguards.

It established a midwife licensing committee and strict guidelines on training and competency standards. License renewal would be required every two years, with evidence to demonstrate that the midwife had been maintaining proper expertise.

The midwife was also required to have a consultive relationship with a physician accorded hospital privileges. In other words, during the rare instance of crisis, a mother could be swiftly transferred to hospital facilities for emergency procedures.

MOST IMPORTANT, the bill would have made good, lasting medical care available to pregnant women who now are unable to get it.

The measure passed the Senate Business and Professions Committee, but unfortunately was voted down by the Appropriations Committee. Senator Killea pledges, nonetheless, to continue to press for midwife licensing, and we offer strong support to her effort. This is an idea whose time has very definitely come. It is good for women and good for babies.

PART FIVE

Epilogue

Chapter 15

MONEY AND POLITICS

A striking feature of postwar Britain was the near universal acclaim for the Labour Party's newly instituted National Health Service. Visiting England in the 1950s, I was surprised to find that even the deepest-dyed Tories welcomed it as a Jolly Good Thing, perhaps because they, too, stood to reap the benefits of free medical and hospital care, available to the entire population without regard to income. As my mother once remarked, 'The rich always like a little bit more.'

An English friend, Julia Werthimer, described her experience of birth *à la* National Health in 1954. She and her husband were both well-paid young professionals; she was a journalist at *Good Housekeeping*, he an executive with the British Film Institute.

'The Health Service was six years old and just getting into its stride. As I was living in London, I was keen to have the baby in a good teaching hospital, one where "natural childbirth" was practised,' Julia said. As soon as her pregnancy was confirmed, she booked into University College Hospital, which arranged for her antenatal visits. 'The second thing I did was to hand a special chit to the milkman which entitled me to a free pint of milk a day during pregnancy and the nursing period.'

During pregnancy she attended the hospital antenatal clinic, first once a month, then fortnightly, and in the final month once a week. The monitoring of the pregnancy was excellent, she said: 'I also attended the natural-childbirth classes during the last months of pregnancy. The influence of Grantly Dick-Read was at its height during those years, and the entire maternity department was run according to his precepts. Husbands were also urged to attend some of the classes, as it was taken for granted that they would be present at the birth.'

At about the seventh month of pregnancy the baby was diagnosed as being in the breech position. Julia was summoned to the hospital so that one of the professors could try to turn it. However, the baby was stuck and the attempt failed. 'I was immediately asked if I would agree to be a case for the medical students at their final exam! I spent a hilarious afternoon being palpated by nervous young students, each trying to worm out of me what the diagnosis really was. Only one of them (a woman, I was glad to see) got it right. For this I was paid five shillings.'

Three weeks before the due date her waters broke, so she rang the hospital and was told to come in. 'I called the ambulance (free, of course), went in, was examined by the obstetrician on duty and told that nothing would happen before morning, so I was tucked into bed with a sedative and my husband went home.'

Two hours later she woke up with 'the most godawful contractions' and was wheeled into the labour room. She had been assured ahead of time that the child would be delivered by one of the teaching staff who was conducting research into breech births: 'Nobody had mentioned, however, that a loud bell would ring throughout the department to announce an unusual birth – so it was a bit of a surprise to find myself lying on my back with my legs wide apart facing a group of students who were thronging in the doorway.'

The birth was short and sharp; her husband never got to the hospital in time. Julia had a total anaesthetic so that the baby could be got out quickly by forceps delivery, and the baby had to go to the premature unit for three days 'because he was somewhat battered. So all my hopes of a natural birth came to naught. But the *care* I received was terrific.'

Also terrific was the social life in the eighteen-bed ward. 'It was great fun being there. We all had our babies in little cribs next to our beds, and talked endlessly about the royal family. There

was a woman doctor whose sole job was to walk the wards showing mothers how to breast-feed. She was known as the "lactation
queen".'

At the time the NHS policy was that every woman should have
her first baby in a hospital, her second and third at home, then back
to the hospital for any subsequent births. As Julia's first birth was
complicated by breech presentation, in 1957 she returned to University College Hospital for her second, when everything went swimmingly. The baby was delivered by a midwife and a medical student;
her husband was there to help administer 'gas-and-air, which you
breathe through a mask'. She also had Pethidine: 'It makes you feel
marvellous, like floating on a pink cloud.'

In 1960 her third and last child was born at home, attended by an
NHS midwife. The routine of antenatal visits, this time at a clinic
staffed by midwives, was much the same. 'A few weeks before the
due date I collected an immense maternity pack (free, of course)
containing everything the midwife would need. The birth was simple,
and my husband was there to give the gas-and-air machine. He was
instructed to bury the placenta in the garden, which should do the
flowers a world of good, the midwife told us. She came every day
for ten days to bathe the baby and take care of me. Altogether, it
was a very relaxed affair, and I was glad that my childbearing days
ended on such a pleasant note.'

By the time Julia Werthimer's grandchild was born in 1990, the
British honeymoon with the National Health Service was long over,
the NHS having been seriously undermined by the notorious cuts
mandated by Margaret Thatcher.

When Julia's daughter-in-law Heti applied to University College
Hospital, which still had the reputation of being in favour of natural
childbirth, she was aghast to find that the hospital now made a
routine practice of rupturing the waters in order to hasten the birth.
On that first visit, Heti was handed a leaflet stating that if the birth
and the baby turned out to be normal, she would be discharged after
six hours, because of shortages of space and staff. She might also
have to endure an electronic foetal monitor – 'I've never met a
mother who didn't find this device unbearable,' Julia told me.

By 1990, home births in England had dwindled to about one per cent, a striking difference from Julia's childbearing days.* Nevertheless, Heti decided to have the baby at home, and engaged a private midwife service which cost a thousand pounds. All went well, with two midwives in attendance throughout a long labour. After the birth the midwives paid twelve more visits to help Heti cope with the unfamiliar job of looking after a new baby.

Unaffected by the Thatcher cuts is an invaluable service provided to all British mothers: a health visitor comes to the house every day for a week after the birth to make sure that all is well, to show the mother how to bathe the baby, and to help her with breast-feeding and any other routine problems. This service exists all over Britain; it has nothing to do with the NHS, but is provided by the local public health authority.

But while the NHS may not seem to be all that it once was, America is still fighting off the merest suggestion of a national health programme; and the spiralling costs of private health care should sound alarm bells for all who doubt the value of Britain's system.

Back in 1950, when Congress was debating President Truman's national health insurance proposal, reproductions of a deeply affecting picture, *The Doctor*, were prominently displayed in thousands of physicians' offices throughout the United States. Painted in the last century by Sir Luke Fildes, *The Doctor* depicted a cluttered Victorian

---

* Sheila Kitzinger sent me the figures for home births in England and Wales from 1927 to 1990. A few examples from the year-by-year list:
    1927: 85 per cent
    1958: 49 per cent
    1970: 13 per cent
    1990: 1 per cent
Her observations as to the reason for the sudden shift since Julia Werthimer's childbearing days:
'Though there is still a statutory requirement to provide a home-birth service, women are warned that it is not safe to give birth outside hospital. Most doctors and the general public have come to believe this without requiring any evidence.
'In 1970 a British Government Committee published the Peel Report, which stated that hospital beds must be provided for all women giving birth. This was accepted as the basis of policy without any evidence, and the maternity services were reorganised around that premise. The views of the women who were using the service were ignored.'

drawing room where a grave-faced physician gazes intently at his small patient, a feverish child, possibly near death. This picture was made the cornerstone of a multimillion-dollar propaganda campaign by the American Medical Association against a universal government insurance plan. The accompanying text delivered the message:

Keep Politics Out of This Picture

When the life – or death – of a loved one is at stake, hope lies in the devoted service of your Doctor. Would you change this picture? Compulsory health insurance is political medicine. It would bring a third party – a politician – between you and your Doctor. It would bind up your family's health in red tape. It would result in heavy payroll taxes – and inferior medical care for you and your family. Don't let that happen here!

Truman's plan was defeated, and subsequent national health insurance bills have all gone down to defeat due to the opposition of the highly financed, ever-watchful physicians' lobby.

The AMA has only had to invoke the dreaded S-word, 'socialised medicine', to send law-makers scurrying for cover and to guarantee a 'no' vote on any such subversive proposal for a fundamental change in the happy doctor–patient relationship.

In 1986, however, two Harvard Medical School professors, Drs Steffie Woolhandler and David Himmelstein, launched Physicians for a National Health Program. Frustrated with the effect of Reaganomics on the nation's health care, they contacted colleagues around the country with their proposal for a national programme akin to that adopted by Canada twenty years earlier.

Here is how the Canadian system works: funded almost entirely by taxes, it covers the country's 26.5 million residents and is administered through the provincial governments. Each resident receives an identification card, which he or she presents when visiting the doctor. The choice of doctor is up to the patient. Services covered include doctor visits, hospital stays, lab tests, surgery, and prenatal care. Doctors do not bill the patient; they send a list of services they've provided each month to the Provincial Health Ministry, which picks up the tab. Nor are Canadians billed for hospitalisation. Each hospital negotiates an annual 'global' budget with the government and pays for operating expenses out of those funds.

An outstanding provision of the Canadian model is its adoption of the single-payer system in which the government, as sole insurer, pays all health-care bills, thus eliminating the multiplicity of administrative costs incurred by competing insurance companies vying with each other for a slice of the lucrative medical pie.

At about the same time that Himmelstein and Woolhandler were at work in Massachusetts gathering adherents for Physicians for a National Health Program, Dr Kevin Grumbach, a specialist in family medicine at the University of California, San Francisco, was plugging away at a similar effort, forming the California Physicians' Alliance, CaPA. He did his family-practice residency at San Francisco General Hospital, which primarily serves the poor and uninsured, 'where it's impossible not to recognise the profound inequities and irrationalities of the US health system. So many of the problems with which I had to contend were beyond an individual physician-patient frame of reference; a lot of the disease was in the system, not just the patient.'

CaPA soon joined forces with PNHP (no point in fretting over these tiresome mazes of initials, as they are part of modern life), which by 1991 had about four thousand dues-paying members in all fifty states. Those members represent a variety of specialities, including academicians, private practitioners, physicians at public clinics – a spectrum of the medical profession.

The initial success of Physicians for a National Health Program in recruiting doctors to its cause should go far to counteract the widely held view of the medical profession as a monolithic mass, uniformly dedicated to the self-serving political and social philosophy of its umbrella organisation and national voice, the American Medical Association. The organisers of PNHP soon discovered that thousands of colleagues around the country are extremely unhappy with the AMA-endorsed status quo and more than ready to break ranks.

On January 12, 1989, Himmelstein and Woolhandler tested their idea for an overhaul of the US health system in an article in the *New England Journal of Medicine* titled 'A National Health Program for the United States: A Physicians' Proposal'. This was followed by their article in the *Journal of General Internal Medicine* of January–February 1989, 'Resolving the Cost/Access Conflict: The Case for a National Health Program'.

With the PNHP in high gear, the American Medical Association felt constrained to go into overdrive, which it did with a packet of information sent in the autumn of 1989 to all US doctors, whether or not members of the 280,000-strong AMA.

The covering letter started: 'Dear Doctor: I have urgent news,' which turned out to be the threat of legislation to 'create a Canadian-type health care system that would hit physicians like you especially hard'. The crux of the letter, set out and underlined:

Our proposal: An intensive program to alert Congress and voters to the dangers of a Canadian-type health care system.

And the punch line:

Take charge of your future by helping us fund the Public Alert Program to strengthen the US health care system. Send your contribution of $200 so we can continue to publish the vital messages in the media.

The vital messages were contained in sample ads, a throwback to that ad showing *The Doctor* of President Truman's day. One showed a wistful little girl and the headline 'In Some Countries She Could Wait Months for Her Surgery', and another depicted an anxious young woman, with the caption 'Elective Surgery: Should it Be Up to You, or a Committee?' The text for each was identical:

We are not talking about life in the Third World.

Some of the most advanced industrial countries on earth have health care systems that are under-financed, overextended and ill equipped.

So what may be routine for us in America can mean an unbearable wait in a system where health care expenditures are controlled by government.

While 'most Americans enjoy the highest quality of health care in the world', and 'without doubt, the US health care system is the finest', the message continued, 'the system is not without its problems'. These, the ad told us, the AMA was working to correct via reform of the Medicaid/Medicare programmes.

Interestingly, the ads nowhere mentioned the 'dangers of a Canadian-type health care system' referred to in the covering letter, possibly because public opinion polls conducted in 1988 by *The Los Angeles Times* and in 1989 by NBC already showed that more than 61 per cent of Americans favoured the Canadian system over that of the United States.

By 1991 *The Wall Street Journal*'s nationwide poll showed that 69 per cent of voters – including 60 per cent of conservatives and 62 per cent of people with household incomes of more than $50,000 – backed such a system, while 20 per cent were opposed.

In its panegyric to the unparalleled excellence of US health care, the AMA neglected to mention some health statistics which should be more than a little embarrassing for the richest nation in the world. On a world scale, the United States' health rankings trail those of Japan, most of the European Community, the Scandinavian countries, Canada, and even Bulgaria and Hong Kong in some categories.

Rankings of the United States among the industrialised nations tell the story:

Life expectancy	12th
Infant mortality	24th
Deaths under 5 years of age	21st
Low birth weight	24th

In 1990 the United States had a total medical bill of $666 billion, or about $2,664 for every man, woman, and child. This is worth pondering, as very few men, women, or children will recall being the beneficiaries of this munificent sum for their medical care. At least 37 million Americans have no health insurance, hence practically no access to health care. The majority of these are not eligible for Medicare or Medicaid because they are families of people who have jobs. For pregnant women who *do* qualify for Medicaid, finding an obstetrician who accepts Medicaid patients is like finding a needle in a haystack. The part-time worker, the minimum-wage earner, the seasonal employee are not legally 'poor', but they can't afford the huge premiums for private health insurance. As of 1991, the price of health premiums had jumped 400 per cent since 1980, with no end in sight.

For the minority who don't have to worry about medical expenses – the affluent, the fully insured, the financially secure retired person – an excursion into the weird and wondrous world of hospital billing systems can help explain the nation's sky-rocketing health bill. Hospital bills are designed, it seems, to confuse, replete with unfamiliar initials and symbols – for example, who knows what Fantanyl In 1M means, priced at $71.48? Or 2Sol IV 1000 ML – $203? 001 Sol IV 1000 ML – $101.50? I plucked these at random from a recent bill issued by Alta Bates Hospital in Berkeley. But we do know what ascorbic acid is – Vitamin C, which can be had in any supermarket for about $2 per 100 pills, or $.02 each. On this bill, they are priced at $3.09 per tablet or, for a total of 22, at $67.98. Multivitamin tablets were $2.79 apiece, seven for $19.53.

Perhaps most of the well-insured hardly bother to read their bills, let alone challenge them – they would leave that to the insurance carrier. As for disputing the charges, the patient unfamiliar with medical terminology wouldn't know where to begin.

One exceptional patient is Dr Ephraim Kahn, a Berkeley specialist in internal medicine. Kahn was admitted to Alta Bates Hospital in August 1991 for three days because of a suspected heart condition. Not one to take things lying down (except under duress, when confined to a hospital bed), Dr Kahn scrutinised his three-day bill as soon as he was up and about and then strode forth to do battle with the billing department.

For the room alone – not in intensive care – the charge was $1,264 per day. Irksome enough, but not in dispute. More of a challenge were charges for 'Partial Bed Bath: $51.52' and 'Complete Bed Bath: $76.71', for a total bathing bill of $128.23. As he had not been favoured with the merest sponge-down, which he would have welcomed during his three-day stay, this seemed a bit absurd. Being a doctor, wise to the ways and jargon of his profession, Dr Kahn noted such items as ten 'Heparin Lock Flush', charged at $13.96 each; only one was done. There was much more, for procedures billed at far over cost or not performed at all.

Dr Kahn described his experience at the billing office. 'It's in a large warehouse type of building about a quarter of a mile from the hospital,' he told me. 'A lady comes out, makes photocopies of the bill which I have brought, and takes notes on my questions. She says she will have an "auditor" go over the bill and will let me know in ten days to two weeks.

'The interesting question is: Why do they bother to make up the bills for Medicare patients? Medicare pays on a DRG basis, meaning Diagnosis Related Group – i.e., they are paid according to the diagnosis, not according to the services rendered in any particular case.'

This may also explain why the normally price-conscious consumer, who would come down hard on overcharges by a department store or a supermarket, ignores unfair billing by a hospital. He or she doesn't have to pay – the bill will ultimately be footed by that faceless entity the taxpayer, or through increased premiums for the insured. Dr Kahn, who does not suffer fools – or knaves, for that matter – gladly, has probably saved a total of $281.90.

Eventually he got one of those mealymouthed letters endemic to the corporate world: 'We are now in the process of adjusting your account. If you have any questions, please feel free to call our business office . . .' and so on. The dénouement is yet to come. The moral, however is clear: None but the brave deserves the fair – hospital bill, that is.

The poshest hospitals, of which Alta Bates is one, are the worst offenders. Cedars-Sinai Medical Center in Los Angeles, which serves the rich and famous – movie stars, network executives, and the like – charged $15 for a pair of disposable paper slippers. Shady Grove Hospital in Rockville, Maryland, charged a patient $11.10 for an item listed as a 'soft foot cast' – actually an elastic bandage for a bruised ankle – and $5.06 for a plastic urine sample cup.

A Los Angeles writer named Joseph Anthony, drawing on testimony provided by a US Senate subcommittee, published these findings in a July 1991 article titled 'Anatomy of a Hospital Bill'. Trying to discover the rationale for such outlandish prices, Anthony noted, 'Hospital administrators usually have a one-word answer handy: "Overhead".' Overhead, it develops, can be construed to cover just about everything, from the cost of the hospital building itself, utilities, staff salaries, medical equipment – depending on the way these items are construed by the accounting department of an individual hospital.

The bills are first examined by the insurance companies and employers, who pay 85 per cent or more of the total cost of hospital care in this country, and who try to keep costs down by ferreting out overcharges. The hospitals then fight back by hiring outside 'revenue-recovery firms' to search out *under*charges. Working on a percentage of the money they recover, these firms zealously encourage employees to seek out undercharges while ignoring overcharges.

One might have thought that this tangled web of deception – hospital and insurance company vying with each other to produce the best and most convincing series of self-serving partial truths, semi-truths, and outright lies – might be a trifle embarrassing to the perpetrators. Not a bit of it. As Dan Hogan, a spokesman for Monongalia General Hospital in Morgantown, West Virginia, explained to Joseph Anthony, 'I know all about these error rates. The average five-day stay here produces a bill with 3,500 line items, and inevitably some of the documentation for a procedure is not going to get done properly, so we're told our bills are inaccurate. A lot of what are called errors are just documentation gaps.'

Similar documentation gaps came under close scrutiny at a hearing of the House Energy and Commerce Committee on July 17, 1991. From bad to worse: where Joseph Anthony had turned up a charge of $1 for a single Tylenol tablet, the committee's investigators chalked up $9 for the same item. Congressman John Dingell of Michigan observed that 'the now famous $640 Pentagon toilet seat pales in the face of some of these hospital charges'. The focus of the investigation, and the source of the statistics on prices, was the Louisville-based Humana Group, one of the largest chains of for-profit 'health-care providers', which then owned seventy-seven hospitals around the country. Committee investigators noted that Humana's policies were typical of hospitals nationwide.

The staff study of billing at Humana's hospitals found that mark-up on supplies averaged 127 per cent. But Bruce F. Chafin, the staff's chief investigator, said that far higher mark-ups were found for some items to which patients pay the least attention. Some examples:

Item	Humana Pays	Patient is Billed
A pair of crutches	$8.35	$103.65
Rubber armpads for crutches	.90	$23.75
Rubber tips for crutches	.71	$15.95
Container of saline solution	.81	$44.90
Heating pad	$5.74	$118.00
Oesophagus tube	$151.98	$1,205.50

Asked to explain, Humana's chairman, David A. Jones, told the House committee that supply costs should not be viewed in isolation because they are adjusted to reflect the total cost of patient care: 'In that context, the true context, they are reasonable and cost-justified,' he said. 'We are not a drugstore. We provide these items as part of the entirety of our patient care and, for better or worse, we price them and charge for them only as an integral component of the total cost of patient care.'

The upshot is that to placate the big insurers, hospitals like the Humana Group – which might be better named Inhumana – have negotiated to reduce room costs in an attempt to bring down overall medical costs, and have shifted overhead costs to supplies. As of 1991, the cost of ancillary supplies and services accounted for about 80 per cent of hospital revenues, while room costs represented only about 20 per cent, a reversal of the ratio of twenty years ago.

And now for the bills behind the bills. We can already glimpse from the foregoing that the lady in the billing office who made photocopies of Dr Kahn's bill, the auditor who would be assiduously auditing his bill, the writer of the letter from Alta Bates business office who was 'in the process of adjusting your account' – each of these must have an office staff, computers, janitors, all the components of efficient business management. Somewhere off in the distance are the outside 'revenue-recovery firms', whose services are paid for by the hospital. Then there are the explainers of bills to the media and Congress – they must command decent salaries, but do not expect them to appear at your hospital bedside with a cold compress for a headache, let alone a bedpan if needed. They are not in business to help or comfort patients, but for a more exalted purpose;

to try to pacify difficult customers like Dr Kahn, to assure assorted legislative committees that the system is working, and to promise dire results if anyone tries to change this best of all possible systems. Above all, these explainers are there to fend off proponents of those hare-brained foreign schemes, alien to all good Americans.

The cost of administering health insurance is so great that it accounts for an estimated 25 cents of every health care dollar.

In one decade, 1975 to 1985, the direct cost just of administering health insurance rose 655 per cent, which accounts in large part for the spectacular rise in the nation's health bill, seen as a percentage of the gross national product:

1966	6.0 per cent
1990	12.4 per cent
1991	13.7 per cent
2000	17.0 per cent*

One obvious reason: in the US there are fifteen hundred different health insurance programmes competing for business, each with its own marketing department, claims processing apparatus, and coverage regulations. Hence an army of accountants, clerical workers with an arsenal of antipersonnel hardware, copying machines and computers, create an avalanche of paperwork, needed to verify in detail what should be paid by various insurers, each with its own rules for coverage. How much for a Band-Aid? An aspirin? Or a pair of disposable paper slippers? Or a nursing bra, charged by Humana at $455? Or, hitting rock bottom, so to speak, one sanitary napkin, priced at $5? That was told to me by a young mother who had given birth in a San Diego hospital. I thought she must be hallucinating until I saw documentation of similar outrageous charges.

In 1991, during the run-up to the November elections, the health crisis first came to a simmer, then to a low boil, and finally began to boil over.

This is due to a new factor emerging in the 1990s. Evidence of the health-care crisis for the *middle* classes mounts daily, in heart-wrenching TV specials showing respectable families of company

* Estimated by the Department of Commerce.

executives forced into bankruptcy because of bills incurred by a devastating illness which the insurance company refused to pay. Politicians who turned a blind eye to the plight of millions of poor people
with no access to decent health care – poor people, after all, have
negligible political influence – are beginning to realise what is happening, when they see statistics like these for 1991 in *The New York
Times*: 'Many people who joined the ranks of the uninsured last year
were relatively affluent. Families with annual incomes of $50,000 or
more accounted for nearly one third of the increase in the number
of people with no health insurance. The number of such uninsured
families with incomes of $50,000 or more rose by 431,000 to a total
of 5.3 million in 1990.' The problem has suddenly moved to the
front burner, thanks to 'the haunting danger of the bourgeois', as
Henry James put it in another context.

By mid-1991 there were no fewer than fourteen congressional
proposals to revamp the nation's health system. Most of these have
not differed markedly from the AMA's 'Health Access America' –
which is not surprising, considering the overwhelming political
power exerted by that organisation via campaign contributions. In
1991, the political watchdog group Common Cause estimated that
political action committees affiliated with the medical industry contributed $60 million to congressional candidates during the last
decade. And the private insurance lobby, which has everything to
gain by sticking with its AMA colleagues, gave over $8.8 million
in campaign contributions in 1990, thus consolidating the lucrative
partnership of fee-for-service medicine and private insurance.

The 'Health Access America' bill's central provision was
employer-mandated health insurance, which would require all busi-
nesses to purchase health insurance for their employees (or to pay a
tax to fund coverage for the uninsured). This, obviously, has nothing
to do with any concept of a universal health care system and everything to do with money and politics.

If America finally adopts this approach to supposedly reforming
its health care system the future for the poor, and for everyone
liable to slip through the net, is bleak indeed; and the likelihood of
humanising childbirth is as remote as ever. Without some form of
single-payer system, and with powerful private interests firmly

entrenched, American women will always be denied the degree of choice which seems possible in Britain and other European countries. In the words of Jennifer Dohrn of Morris Heights, American women will go on being delivered of their babies and never be allowed the experience of *giving* birth to them.

ACKNOWLEDGMENTS

As everyone knows, the normal duration of pregnancy for a human is nine months. As some of us thought we knew (having been told this as children), for an elephant it takes twice as long – eighteen months. 'Oh poor her!' we would exclaim, thinking about the dear elephant and her suffering. For dinosaurs, nobody really knows at this late date. Possibly three or four years? If so, this book is dinosaur progeny.

During its long gestation, I sought the help of numerous experts in this country and abroad – doctors, midwives, nurses, public health workers, lawyers, mothers – many of whom contributed invaluable information, and are duly credited in the text.

There are others to whom I am greatly indebted. Renée Wayne Golden, a Hollywood lawyer who specialises in entertainment law, is my literary representative and in many ways the fairy godmother of this book. She urged me to write it in the first place, and as time went on was a fund of useful suggestions. Although it's not exactly 'entertainment', – who knows? Given her specialised talents she may yet sell the musical comedy rights to some Broadway producer, if one could only think of a catchy title. *Les Mids? Oh! Cal Cut Her!* (in which Dr Cal performs a Caesarean to the background music of 'I've got you under my skin . . .')? *A Chorus Line* (featuring the top brass of the American Medical Association singing 'Oh no, You can't take that away from me')?

I first met William Abrahams, editor extraordinaire, when he turned up in northern California as West Coast editor of the *Atlantic Monthly*. As an occasional writer for the mag, I was amazed and delighted at the amount of time he put in meticulously editing and greatly improving my articles. Thus it was a joy to find out that he would be my editor for *The American Way of Birth*. At the slightest moan from me, Billy would come springing up from Hillsborough – a good hour's drive – and help to unscramble a messy bit of manuscript, or to show the way out of that unhappy condition known as Writer's Block.

As for my assistant Catherine Edwards, who has helped me in all my endeavours – articles, books, etc. – over many years, she is not only extremely clever and skilful at everything she puts her hand to, but she is great fun to work with. I am not sure, however, if she got much pleasure out of this particular job. One morning she arrived to find next to her typewriter a huge tome, *Williams Obstetrics*, which I had inadvertently left open at a particularly revolting anatomical drawing of an episiotomy. 'Who'd ever want to have a baby after reading *your* book!' she exclaimed.

For research assistance, I must thank first and foremost Ted Kalman, who worked with me from the beginning, helped to clarify the approach to various subjects – especially the midwife aspects, on which he is extremely knowledgeable – and who arranged innumerable appointments to which he accompanied me with his trusty tape recorder. He read the manuscript in various stages and made many needed changes.

Travelling from California to Washington, Atlanta, and Montgomery in pursuit of information, I knew that I would be needing in each of these far-away cities what politicians call an 'advance man' to line up appointments and ferry me from hither to yon. Thanks to the kindness of strangers, I could not have wished for better guidance from the following:

Washington. Dana Hughes, who had worked in the national office of the Children's Defense Fund; her husband Daniel Lindheim, former aide to Congressman Ron Dellums; and Roberta Brooks of Dellums's Oakland headquarters. Wise in the ways of the nation's capital, they provided entrée to some of the principal wheelers and dealers in the maternity-care scene, from politicians to heads of national professional associations. They clued me in to which agencies would be useful and which to avoid. Best of all, they put me in touch with the ideal guide to that mystifying city: Gawain Kripke, who lined up our schedule, spent many days driving me from office to office, and was an invaluable participant in discussions with all and sundry.

Atlanta. My daughter Constancia Romilly, a nurse in the county hospital, swung straight into action to line up an advance man – in this case, an advance woman, Betty Corbett, herself in a fairly advanced stage of pregnancy. Between them, they mapped out an itinerary including a visit to Ina May Gaskin at The Farm. My thanks to them, and congratulations to Betty, who despite (or perhaps because of) arduous driving round the area gave birth to the Perfect Baby shortly thereafter.

Montgomery. For an introduction to the innovative Gift of Life program, I am indebted to Virginia Durr, a native of that city with rare insight into the intricacies of Alabama politics. She arranged for a young public health worker Dawn Cox to show me around. My thanks to them.

An enjoyable detour was afforded by my efforts to find out a bit more about Queen Victoria's interesting addiction to 'blessed chloroform'. This is mentioned glancingly in biographies by Stanley Weintraub and others, but surely the Queen, a prolific letter-writer, would have had more to say on the subject? I shall ever cherish the memory of this particular search, which went something like this:

1) I consult Professor Peter Stansky of the Stanford University History Department.

2) He recommends Professor Kenneth Bourne of the London School of Economics & Political Science.

3) Professor Bourne advises writing to 'The Librarian, Mr Oliver Everett, Windsor Castle, Berkshire'.

4) I do so, and I am rewarded with everything the heart could desire – diaries and notes from the Queen's doctors, plus photocopies of some of her unpublished letters on the subject. But oh! her hand-writing – atrocious, due no doubt to the teachings of her ghastly German governess Baroness Lehzen. I could barely decipher one word in five.

5) Back to Professor Stansky, who turned the project over to Professor Carolyn Lougee and graduate students in British history at

Stanford. Thanks to them, this minuscule slice of history is now preserved.

Finally, my profound thanks to the following for their time, help, and invaluable expertise:

Midwives: Educators Suzanne Arms and Elizabeth Davis, writers whose books I had read and admired, who helped fill me in with further information. Also, many members of the Midwives' Alliance of North America and members of the California Association of Midwives with whom I met on several occasions over the past few years and whose dedication to their calling – and courage in face of attack – is a rare pleasure to behold.

Researcher: Rachel Stocking, graduate student at Stanford University, who fetched up quick as a wink articles from medical journals and prepared synopses of them.

Typists: Stenotypist Katherine Lauster who transcribed myriad tapes; Rachel Stocking who wore two hats: expert researcher and typist; and Susan MacCulloch who came in for the kill, just at deadline, to finish typing the manuscript with rare speed and accuracy.

Volunteer readers: Friends and relations on whom I inflicted chunks of book-in-progress, and who sustained me with help and advice: Shana Alexander, Marge Frantz and her daughter Virginia, Sally Belfrage, Bob Treuhaft, the pseudonymous Mary Welcome, Cynthia and Roy Campbell, and Constancia Romilly – who is, in fact, the 'C. R.' of Chapter 13, Morris Heights.

J. M.
March 1, 1992

SOURCE NOTES

Chapter 2: A GLANCE BACKWARD

page

24 All quotations from *Malleus Maleficarum* are from the translation by Montague Summers (London: The Fortune Press, 1948).

26 'but one female inhabitant each' Barbara Ehrenreich and Deirdre English, *For Her Own Good* (New York: Doubleday Anchor, 1979), p. 35.
    'more recent assessments' Robert Bartlett, *New York Review of Books*, 13 June 1991.

28 'gowns of rich stuff' *Encyclopedia Britannica*.
    'which members were obliged to attend' *Dictionary of the Middle Ages*.

29 'cupped the baby's head' Richard W. Wertz and Dorothy C. Wertz, *Lying-In: A History of Childbirth in America* (New York: Schocken Books, 1979), p.35.
    'banging with hammers during the delivery' This account drawn from Anthony Smith, *The Body* (New York: Viking, 1986), p. 54.

31 'to which by Oath he is bound' Irving S. Cutter, *A History of Midwifery*; and (with Henry R. Viets) *A Short History of Midwifery* (Philadelphia: Saunders, 1964).
    'Arbiters of Life and Death' Cutter, op. cit., p. 50.
    'speaking most of the languages' Cutter, op. cit., p. 51.

32 'the negotiations are very obscure' Logan Clendening, *The Romance of Medicine* (Garden City, NY: Garden City Publishing Co., 1933), p. 150.
    'presented to the Medico-Chirurgical Society' Cutter, op. cit., p. 50.
    'both of Woman and Child' Cutter, op. cit., p. 55.

33 'not a single death from the fever' Clendening, op. cit., p. 330.

34 'This disease did not exist in the town' Clendening, op. cit.
    'its ravages were equally striking' Clendening, op. cit.

35 'even with the aid of repeating washing' Cutter, op. cit., p. 116.

36 'an all-important discovery' Cutter, op. cit.
    'became ill with the fever' Wertz and Wertz, op. cit., p. 121.

37 'happy in ignorance of danger' Wertz and Wertz, op. cit., p. 122.
    'clean hands can carry the disease' Wertz and Wertz, op. cit., p. 123.

38 'marched up to support my position' Cutter, op. cit., p. 135.

39 'the sense of delicacy, on the part of the female' in *Obstetrical Catechism* (1854), quoted in Wertz and Wertz, op. cit., p. 83.

40 'will not be flurried or shocked' Wertz and Wertz, op. cit., pp. 83–84.
'the second wealthiest of all American doctors' I am indebted in the paragraphs that follow for a vivid account of Sims's career in G. J. Barker-Benfield, *The Horrors of the Half-Known Life* (New York: Harper & Row, 1976), Chapter 10 'Architect of the Vagina'.

42 'anaesthetic properties of chloroform' Eve Blantyre Simpson, *Sir James Y. Simpson* (New York: Scribners, 1896).
'choke him off the pursuit' Simpson, op. cit.

43 'in time of trouble for help' Mary Poovey, *Uneven Developments* (Chicago: University of Chicago Press, 1988).
'Queen Victoria had been interested' The account of the Queen and 'blessed chloroform' has been made possible by the generous assistance of the Librarian of Windsor Castle, as described in my Acknowledgments, pp. 223–4.

45 'meddlesome midwifery' Quoted in Wertz and Wertz, op. cit., and Poovey, op. cit.

47 'subsequent improvements were offshoots' The account of the first Caesarean is drawn from Wertz and Wertz, op. cit., p. 139.

48 'close to 100 per cent' Wertz and Wertz, op. cit., pp. 132–5.

Chapter 3: FASHIONS IN CHILDBIRTH

52 'Twilight Sleep Association' Again I am indebted to Wertz and Wertz, pp. 150–2.

53 'extensively employed here and abroad' Joseph B. DeLee, *The Principles and Practice of Obstetrics* (Philadelphia: W. B. Saunders, 1940).

55 'an animal howling in pain' Sheila Kitzinger, *The Complete Book of Pregnancy and Childbirth* (New York: Alfred A. Knopf, 1985) p. 241.

57 'ether-paraldehyde oil' DeLee, op. cit.
'will spontaneously disappear' DeLee, op. cit.

61 'labour without pain' Fernand Lamaze, *Painless Childbirth* (Chicago: Henry Regnery, 1970).

63 'a refinement of cruelty' Leboyer quotations are from *The New Our Bodies, Ourselves* (Boston Women's Health Book Collective, 1984). Other books consulted for accounts of Bradley and Leboyer are Margot Edwards and Mary Waldorf, *Reclaiming Birth*; Kitzinger, *The Complete Book of Pregnancy and Childbirth*, and Wertz and Wertz, *Lying-In*.

64 'The house bought drinks back' Warren Hinckle, 'Fifty-something', *San Francisco Examiner*, 3 December 1989.
'giggling girlishly' Hinckle, op. cit.

65 'waving and flapping in the air' Hinckle, op. cit.

66 '*The Birth Gazette*' Quarterly publication, The Farm, Summertown, TN, 38483.
'the option of using the cushion' *Independent*, London, 7 July 1989.

68 'Writs of Habeas Foetus' *San Francisco Chronicle*, 4 August 1989.

Chapter 4: THE IMPOVERISHED WAY

70 'infant mortality' California Physicians Alliance Workshop Newsletter, November 1990.
'*Babies at Risk*' 'Frontline', produced for WGBH, Boston, 1989.

Chapter 5: OBSTETRICIANS

87 'an interesting series of index entries' J. Whitridge Williams, *Williams Obstetrics*, 18th ed. (East Norwalk, Conn.; Appleton & Lang, 1989).

87– 'During the mid-1970s Diana Scully' Quotes from interviews at 'Elite
70 Medical Center', from Diana Scully, *Men Who Control Women's Health: The Miseducation of Obstetrician-Gynecologists* (Boston: Houghton Mifflin, 1980).

93 'OB/GYN practitioners will be women' American College of Obstetricians and Gynecologists, *Women in Obstetrics/Gynecology*, 3 January 1991, Table III.

95 '"accept me as an equal person," she wrote' *San Francisco Chronicle*, 4 June 1991.
'run his hand up my leg' *San Francisco Examiner*, 9 June 1991.

96 'slide on breasts never appeared again' *San Francisco Examiner*, 9 June 1991.

Chapter 6: ELECTRONIC FOETAL MONITORS AND ULTRASOUND

101 'Whither Electronic Monitoring?' *Obstetrics and Gynecology*, vol. 76, no. 6 (December 1990).

102 'rather than an electronic monitor' Paul B. Coditz and David J. Henderson-Smart, *Medical Journal of Australia*, vol. 153 (1990), p. 88, quoted in *Physiology of Pregnancy, Labor and Puerperim*.

103 'suffer delayed effects in later life' Kitzinger, op. cit., p. 185.
'As for its diagnostic usefulness' *Obstetrics and Gynecology*, vol. 76, no. 2 (August 1990).

104 'published its findings the following year' Royal Society of Medicine (London), *Birth*, vol. 13, Special Supplement (December 1986).
'may be harmful to mother and child' Ann Oakley's footnotes cite the source as F. J. Browne, ed., *Antenatal and Postnatal Care*, 2nd ed. (London: J. & A. Churchill, 1937), p. 497; and 9th ed. (1960), p. 389.
'without the use of diagnostic ultrasound' Oakley's sources: L. N. Reece, *Proceedings of the Royal Society of Medicine 1935*, vol. 18, p. 489; and S. N. Hassani, *Ultrasound in Gynecology and Obstetrics* (New York: Springer-Verlag, 1978), p. vii.

Chapter 7: FORCEPS

107 'they murder twenty'   *American Journal of Obstetrics and Gynecology*, vol. 145 (March–April 1983).

109 'Midforceps Delivery – a Vanishing Art?'   David N. Danforth and Averon Ellis, *American Journal of Obstetrics and Gynecology*, vol. 86 (1963): 29.

110 'voluntary cooperation of the patient'   L. V. Dill, *The Obstetrical Forceps* (Springfield, Ill.: Charles Thomas, 1953).

111 'Can Mid-Forceps Operations Be Eliminated?'   *Obstetrics and Gynecology*, vol. 2 (1953): 302.

112 'not according to what we did'   *Contemporary OB/GYN*, vol. 15 (May 1980).

113 'may perform thirty to forty each year'   'Current Role of the Midforceps Operation', Watson A. Bowles and Christine Bowes, *Clinical Obstetrics and Gynecology*, vol. 23, no. 2 (June 1980).

'symposium documented in May 1980'   *Contemporary OB/GYN*, vol. 15 (May 1980).

Chapter 8: CAESAREANS

115 'only released two years later – in July 1991'   *San Francisco Chronicle*, from Medical Tribune Service, 11 July 1991.

117 'which will need antibiotic treatment'   Mortimer Rosen, *The Cesarean Myth* (New York: Viking, 1989), p. 21.

'back to normal after six weeks'   Lynn Silver and Sidney M. Wolfe, *Unnecessary Cesarean Sections: How to Cure a National Epidemic* (Public Citizen Health Research Group, 1989).

120 'preparing for future births'   *Birthways*, Cesarean Prevention Movement of San Diego newsletter, Sept–Oct 1991.

121 'induction of labour, and VBACs'   In *Mothering* (summer 1989), article by Josala A. Ferherolf.

'beautiful prose along the same lines'   *Birthways* (Sept–Oct 1991).

122 'including learning disabilities'   Don Creevy, chapter in *Learning Disabilities and Prenatal Risk* (Urbana and Chicago: University of Illinois Press, 1986).

123 'maternal mortality in Rhode Island'   Evrard and Gold, *Obstetrics and Gynecology*, vol. 50 (1977): 594–7.

'including hysterectomy and bowel trauma'   Institute of Medicine, *Medical Professional Liability and the Delivery of Obstetrical Care*, vol. 1 (Washington, DC: National Academy Press, 1989): 76.

124 'undermining the teaching and training of medical students'   Institute of Medicine, op. cit.

'know-how in managing vaginal breech delivery'   Don Creevy, personal communication, September 1991.

126 'too small for a normal birth'   Mortimer Rosen op. cit., p. 24; and Don Creevy, personal communication.

'inadequate uterine or other muscular activity'   Sally B. Olds, Marcia L.

London, and Patricia Ladewig, *Maternal-Newborn Nursing* (Massachusetts: Addison-Wesley, 1984), p. 1028.

'As described by Dr Mortimer Rosen' In *The Cesarean Myth*, op. cit.

128 'it's time to go to the hospital' Nancy Cohen and Lois J. Estner, *Silent Knife* (South Hadley, Massachusetts: Bergin & Garvey, 1983), p. 19.

'poor progress in active labor' National Institute of Child Health and Human Development, National Institutes of Health, draft report of the Task Force on Cesarean Childbirth, September 1980.

129 'for every infant with real foetal distress' Silver and Wolfe, *Unnecessary Cesarean Sections*, op. cit., p. 19.

132 'accounts for 90 per cent of private clinic births' Warren Pearse, personal communication, 9 April 1990.

'honeymoon fresh' *Independent*, London, 4 February 1992.

'who receive a fee for services' Jane Brody, Personal Health column, *New York Times*, 27 July 1989.

133 'differences in clinical management' Jeffrey B. Gould, Becky Davey, and Randall Stafford, 'Socioeconomic Differences in Rates of Caesarean Section', *New England Journal of Medicine* (27 July 1989).

'problems during vaginal births' Daniel Haney (Associated Press), *Montgomery Advertiser*, 27 July 1989.

134 'one of Georgia's lowest rates – 18.7 per cent' *Atlanta Journal and Constitution*, 27 January 1989.

136 'a third to a half of the amount awarded' Statistics available from the American College of Obstetricians and Gynecologists, 409 Twelfth St, Washington, DC, 20024–2188.

137 'plaintiffs do not usually win' Quoted in Patricia Danzon, *Medical Malpractice* (Cambridge: Harvard University Press, 1985).

'compensation via the malpractice system' Victoria Rostow (director, Institute of Medicine), *Medical Professional Liability and the Delivery of Obstetrical Care* (Washington, DC: National Academy Press, 1989), 2 vols.

138 'the threat of malpractice litigation' Ephraim Kahn, personal communication, 6 October 1991.

140 'diagnostic and monitoring procedures' Institute of Medicine, Report, 1989.

'which generally follows the major insurers' lead' Institute of Medicine, Report, 1989.

Chapter 9: IN SEARCH OF MIDWIVES

146 'getting nurse-midwife care' *Nurse-Midwifery in America*, report of the American College of Nurse-Midwives Foundation, 1522 K St, NW, Washington, DC, 20005, 1986.

149 'feelings which are passionate and basic' *Independent*, London, 19 October 1988, quotation from Kitzinger, *The Midwife Challenge*.

Chapter 11: CERTIFIED NURSE-MIDWIVES

158 'set forth in *Nurse-Midwifery in America*'   Report of the American College of Nurse-Midwives Foundation, 1986.

159 'heavily on the side of the midwives'   *Nurse-Midwifery in America*, op. cit.

Chapter 12: THE FARM

168 Ina May Gaskin, *Spiritual Midwifery* (Summertown, Tennessee: The Book Publishing Co., 1975).

169 'for the Haight-Ashbury hippie crowd'   *Tennessee Illustrated*, January 1989; *Atlanta Journal and Constitution*, 23 April, 1989.

174 Helen Varney, *Nurse-Midwifery*, 2nd ed. (Oxford: Blackwell Scientific, 1987).

175 'to the level of the brute creation'   Quoted in Poovey, op. cit., p. 30.

Chapter 14: MIDWIVES UNDER THE GUN

189 'regional enforcement committees'   Julianne D'Angelo, supervising attorney, Center for Public Interest Law, telephone interview with the author, 20 October 1990.

191 'I hope this court will take the opportunity'   From the transcript of the trial.

192 'in-depth look at its procedures'   From the transcript of the trial.

195 'You are prepared for the worst'   *Sacramento Bee*, and *Sacramento Union*, 10 April 1990.

Chapter 15: MONEY AND POLITICS

209 'ever-watchful physicians' lobby'   Kevin Grumbach, 'Seminars in Health Care Delivery.' *Western Journal of Medicine*, 1989.

210 'operating expenses out of those funds'   Constance Matthiessen, staff writer at the Center for Investigative Reporting in San Francisco, *Washington Post*, 27 November 1990.

212 'backed such a system'   *Wall Street Journal*, 28 June 1991.

  'low birth weight . . . 24th'   Statistics from Health Access Foundation, 1535 Mission St, San Francisco, CA 94103 (April 1991).

214 'A Los Angeles writer'   *San Francisco Chronicle*, 14 July 1991; 'Anatomy of a Hospital Bill' by Joseph Anthony, reprinted from *In Health Magazine*.

216 'total cost of patient care'   Douglas Frantz, *Los Angeles Times*, quoted in *San Francisco Chronicle*, 18 October 1991.

218 'a total of 5.3 million in 1990'   Robert Pear, quoting Center for National Health Program Studies, Harvard Medical School, in *New York Times*, 19 December 1991.

  'fee-for-service medicine and private insurance'   Report from Health Access Foundation, op. cit.

INDEX